A MANUAL OF OPERATING ROOM TECHNOLOGY

Frances Ginsberg, R.N., M.S.

Consultant in Aseptic Practice, Bingham Associates Fund, Tufts–New England Medical Center, Boston, Mass.; Formerly Instructor, Operating Room Nursing, Yale University School of Nursing, New Haven, Conn.; Assistant Professor, Operating Room Nursing, Boston University School of Nursing, Boston, Mass.

Lillian Sholtis Brunner, R.N., M.S.

Instructor, Operating Room Nursing, Bryn Mawr Hospital School of Nursing, Bryn Mawr, Pa. Formerly Assistant Professor Surgical Nursing, Yale University School of Nursing, New Haven, Conn. Operating Room Supervisor, Hospital of the University of Pennsylvania, Philadelphia, Pa.

Vernita L. Cantlin, R.N., M.S.

Consultant in Operating Room Nursing, Bryn Mawr, Pa. Formerly Assistant Director of Nursing and Director of the Operating Room, The Chester County Hospital, West Chester, Pa. Operating Room Supervisor, The Graduate Hospital of the University of Pennsylvania, Philadelphia, Pa.

Foreword by

Alfred Hurwitz, M.D.

Director of Surgical Services, Mount Sinai Hospital, Miami Beach, Florida; Formerly Professor of Surgery, State University of New York, College of Medicine. Associate Clinical Professor of Surgery, Yale University School of Medicine

A MANUAL OF
OPERATING ROOM TECHNOLOGY

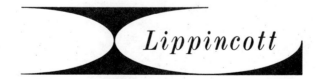

J. B. LIPPINCOTT COMPANY
PHILADELPHIA · TORONTO

Distributed in Great Britain by

Blackwell Scientific Publications, Oxford, London, and Edinburgh

Library of Congress Catalog Card Number: 66–17293

ISBN-0-397-54052-3

Printed in the United States of America

11   12   10

PREFACE

The operating room technician has rather rapidly become an essential and accepted member of an operating room team. Various names have been conferred on these relatively new workers. The list includes nursing assistants, surgical technicians and surgical technical aides. Each of these titles should imply a trained and educated lay person who, following a well-planned program of instruction which combines theory and practice, is prepared to provide a valuable service to the professional nursing staff in the operating room, the patient, the surgeon and the anesthesiologist. Within the past few years the position and preparation of the operating room technician have been studied and carefully scrutinized by many groups representing both nursing and medicine. The result is that today a fairly concise picture of his/her role can be presented. In hospitals throughout the country the course of study designed to prepare this person has shown wide disparity in terms of its nature, content, methods and length.

This book is an attempt to establish content in line with essential and realistic objectives. Content has been delineated and clarified to emphasize principles and to direct the learner toward sound application of these truths. Even though principles are stressed, many of the details of application have not been included inasmuch as they vary from one operating room to another. Then, too, most instructors appreciate optimum latitude in adapting theory to practice. This, we believe, is desirable, since a more meaningful learning experience as well as a higher level of achievement results than would be acquired through a stereotyped general course. It is our contention that the best learning situation exists in or very near the operating room with a prepared and enthusiastic instructor present to guide, teach, demonstrate, answer questions, stimulate interest, provide moral support and utilize the rich resources of the hospital setting.

Since better learning occurs in a "real" environment, we have not included illustrations of instruments, instrument setups and common equipment; these are readily available in every operating room. Handling, using, noting characteristics and unusual qualities of various pieces of equipment increases a learner's under-

v

standing, thoughtful care and use of equipment far more effectively than does leafing through a book of pictures. It must be emphasized, however, that illustrations do serve an important role. A well-chosen picture focuses the learner's attention on a particular feature, a demonstrated principle, or a useful technic far more effectively and quickly than does a descriptive paragraph. Therefore, while being discriminatory, we have been generous in using meaningful illustrations.

Considerable thought has been given to presenting content in well-organized units. Consequently, Unit 1 is an orientation to operating room technology. Here a brief history and description of operating room practice precede the objectives of a program in operating room technology. This is followed by a description of kinds of hospitals and their organizational patterns. Then a similar approach to the operating room and its personnel is given.

Unit 2 presents the fundamental principles and practices of surgical asepsis, including microbiology, human body defenses, sterilization and disinfection. Further expansion and application of these principles continue in subsequent chapters, along with the preparation of personnel and supplies.

The reason for the existence of an operating room is the patient undergoing surgery. Unit 4, therefore, is concerned with the physical and mental preparation of the patient, as well as the safe and complete preparation of the total environment in which the patient will receive the anesthetic agent and submit to the operation. Records relevant to patient care also are described.

The nature and procedures involved in an operation are found in Unit 4. First, a detailed word picture of the usual procedure in a surgical operation is given. Then, ten common operations are described. When the student has acquired understanding and satisfactory performance in assisting with these operations, he is able to adapt or transfer his learning, adding modifications peculiar to other types of surgery, such as neurosurgery, lung or heart surgery.

Care of the patient subsequent to the operation is continued in Unit 5. This includes the terminal care of the operating room and the disposition of all supplies and equipment.

The last unit, Unit 6, presents problem situations and responsibilities, such as those having legal implications or those of an emergency nature. Our premise is that the student must be taught the limitations of his new role as well as the details of his job description.

Following each chapter are a bibliography and a set of review questions.

We gratefully acknowledge the assistance of Earle H. Spaulding, Ph.D., Chief of the Department of Microbiology, Temple University School of Medicine, Philadelphia, Pa., for his suggestions regarding the section on chemical disinfection and sterilization. We are indebted also to David T. Miller and Barton H. Lippincott of the J. B. Lippincott Company for their encouragement and assistance.

FRANCES GINSBERG
LILLIAN SHOLTIS BRUNNER
VERNITA L. CANTLIN

FOREWORD

The authors of this book have made a major contribution to surgery. As surgeons, we have for a long time recognized the need for technologists trained in operating room technics not only because of the paucity of scrub nurses with special training but also because properly trained operating room technologists have been of inestimable value in performing the duties of a scrub nurse. Since the advisability of assigning technologists to our surgical teams is evident, it behooves us to make sure that they are well grounded in basic principles and capable of executing their responsibilities in a highly satisfactory manner. The *Manual of Operating Room Technology* is a milestone in the development of this new field of endeavor.

The authors have gone to great pains to describe not only *what* should be done but, more important, *why* it should be done. The chapters are concise yet meaty, and replete with explanatory statements and much factual knowledge. The chapters deal with the principles and practices of surgical asepsis; preparation and specific responsibilities of operating room personnel; the surgical patient, including his preoperative anxieties; some of the technics employed in the operating room; and postoperative care. The discussions on methods of sterilization and the advantages and disadvantages of various methods and antiseptic agents are especially illuminating and thought-provoking. The final chapters on medicolegal implications and responsibilities and on emergency situations reveal a thoughtful approach to these problems. The book is well illustrated. I learned many new concepts in the perusal of this book and would recommend it most highly to operating room and recovery room nurses, as well as to nursing students, residents and members of the surgical staff, especially those who are members of the operating room committee.

Miss Ginsberg, Mrs. Brunner and Mrs. Cantlin have succeeded beautifully in producing a "Bible" not only for aspiring surgical technologists, but also for the graduate nurse and professional personnel interested in their development. This book should grace the shelves of all hospital and operating room libraries and should be made mandatory reading for all students embarking on careers as operating room technologists or as operating room nurses.

ALFRED HURWITZ, M.D.

CONTENTS

ix

UNIT 3. THE SURGICAL PATIENT

UNIT 4. SURGICAL PROCEDURES

UNIT 1

Orientation to the Operating Room

CHAPTER 1

THE BROAD VIEW OF OPERATING ROOM TECHNOLOGY

INTRODUCTION : A BRIEF HISTORY OF SURGERY AND ASEPSIS :
MODERN PROGRESS : THE TEAM SPIRIT : THE OPERATING ROOM
OF TODAY : OBJECTIVES OF A PROGRAM IN OPERATING ROOM
TECHNOLOGY

INTRODUCTION

One of the best places to observe some of the miracles of the present Golden Age of medical progress is in the operating room of almost any modern hospital. In a way, looking into today's surgical department is an experience very much like the one that Alice in Wonderland must have had when she looked in amazement through the giant glass. In order to understand better the development of modern surgery, let us imagine that Alice had a twin set of glasses through which we, too, can see far into the past as well as through the walls of today's typical operating room.

A BRIEF HISTORY OF SURGERY AND ASEPSIS

Surgery is a type of medical practice in which disease is cured and deformities are corrected by means of manual operative procedures. The sharpened flint probably was one of the first instruments used before the dawn of civilization. In ancient India the famous writing, the *Samhita,* gives a clear-cut classification of surgical operations. In Greece (400 B.C.) Hippocrates knew and described surgical conditions varying from a clubfoot to a fracture of the vertebra. Through the centuries

3

relatively little progress was made in surgical practice because of three major problems: (1) pain, (2) bleeding and (3) infection. (Fig. 1)

Pain. For a long time alcohol and opium were used to lessen surgical pain, but a relatively safe and effective anesthetic agent was not known before 1842, when Dr. Crawford W. Long, of Athens, Georgia, first used ether. In 1846 William T. G. Morton, a Boston dentist, gave the first public demonstration of the use of ether as an anesthetic agent. Then chloroform was introduced, but because of its toxic effects it was later abandoned in this country. It was not until the late 1940's that departments of anesthesiology were set up in medical schools and equipped with research facilities; in its own right this field became an important medical specialty. Today, without the skill of the anesthesiologist, the refined preanesthetic medications, and the available anesthetics, extensive and radical surgery could not be performed safely.

Hemorrhage. Ancient Greeks and Romans used ligatures (strings to tie bleeding blood vessels) to stop hemorrhage following the amputation of extremities. In the Middle Ages this practice was replaced by the use of a hot iron or cautery. In the 16th century a French Army surgeon, Ambroise Paré revived and popularized the ligature. However, it was not until the 20th century that a wide variety of strong and relatively inert sutures and ligatures became available. These include metals, synthetics, silk, cotton and surgical gut.

Infection. Not until the middle of the 19th century was it proved by many scientists that infection is caused by bacteria (germs). The greatest of this group was Louis Pasteur, a French chemist and microbiologist. During this period an English surgeon, Joseph Lister, was the first (1865) to apply this knowledge to the treatment of wounds. By the use of such antiseptics as carbolic acid (phenol) he showed that wound infection could be reduced. This discovery ushered in the era of asepsis—that is, modern surgery without infection.

MODERN PROGRESS

Our own century is filled with dramatic advances. New knowledge in the field of physiology led to a better understanding of fluid balance in the body and its relationship to health and disease. In the field of anesthesia the introduction of positive pressure devices, intratracheal tubes, better preoperative medicine, and antibiotics and the lowering of body temperature have permitted surgeons to enter the heart, to repair the lungs and to treat the brain.

Modern operating rooms now have a variety of monitoring devices which are used to show graphically the living rhythms of the body. Synthetic or plastic replacements and transplanted organs are becoming more commonplace. The highest quality of preoperative preparation, surgical skill and recovery room care, followed by individualized rehabilitation, is available today for most surgical patients. Continued research and advances are being made, which make the operating room one of the most fascinating and dramatic of all places to work.

THE TEAM SPIRIT

Of utmost importance in the successful conduct of operating room activities is the cooperative team spirit within the members of the operating personnel. The contribution of each person is like the links of a chain—the continuity and the strength of each part are vital to its existence. The critical thinking and judgment of leaders are respected and followed. In such a working situation the range of emotions one experiences is considerable—the deep satisfaction when surgery can help a person, or the feeling of great helplessness when a diseased body is beyond the help of the operating team. In the operating room one is aware of the presence of a power greater than man. Here one soon acquires the feeling that the greatest satisfaction from work comes when that work is related to serving those who cannot help themselves.

THE OPERATING ROOM OF TODAY

Now let us focus our attention on specific aspects of the operating room.

The Patient. Every kind of person can be seen as a patient in the operating room: the richest, the poorest, the wisest, the dullest, the best known, the unknown, the tallest, the smallest, the oldest, the youngest. And yet every one is received in the

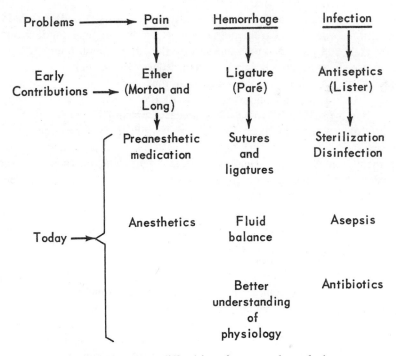

Fig. 1. Overcoming three difficulties of surgery through the years.

operating room as an individual who has certain rights and needs. He is treated with kindness, dignity and respect. He may have only a tiny mole removed, or he may have a badly battered and burned body in need of extensive repair. Whoever works in the operating room is expected to care for every patient as if he, the worker, were the patient.

Environment. It is a well-known fact that germs cause infection and disease. The success of any operation in large measure depends on the removal from the wound site and the surrounding area of as many disease-producing organisms as is humanly possible. This means that everything in the operating room must be thoroughly clean, and this standard includes healthy personnel. One sneeze from a person who has a cold may be all that is necessary to infect an open wound. Clothing must be clean. Walls, ceilings, floors, tables, lamps, cupboards, etc., must be free of dust, dirt, lint and debris. Movement of personnel, conversation and the opening of doors, all help to dispense increasing numbers of organisms in air currents; therefore, limitations in all of these activities are necessary for their control. Those articles and pieces of equipment that can be sterilized are made free of organisms. In most operating rooms the ventilation system is such that air pressure is increased to prevent the entrance of dust particles through an open door. Some specially constructed rooms even are equipped with a higher than atmospheric concentration of oxygen (these are called hyperbaric chambers) and are used for special surgical conditions.

Instruments, Machines and Equipment. In addition to the scalpel, which is the surgeon's knife, one sees a tremendous variety of instruments made from many kinds of metals and plastics. Some are so tiny that the surgeon requires a magnifying lens to use them effectively in very small body cavities, such as the middle ear. Some pieces of equipment are so large that they occupy a large section of the operating room and actually take over part of the patient's normal function. An example is the heart-lung machine. This piece of machinery carries on the pumping and the oxygenation of the patient's blood while the surgeon repairs a defect in the heart.

Instruments come in many shapes and sizes, depending on their use. Some resemble carpenters' tools; others, small sewing machines, miniature garden tools, telescopic equipment, barber and dental aids. Many are unusually strange, designed for certain relatively rare jobs. Each instrument was created and designed for a particular purpose and must be used that way. You will share in the responsibility of caring for, cleaning and handling these instruments, many of which cost hundreds and even thousands of dollars.

Personnel. So many of the activities that once belonged to man—farming, road building, mathematical computation and dress making, to mention a few—now are taken over completely by machines. Repairing the human body is one activity that seems safe from the complete domination of a machine. Human beings and their services to other human beings are the heart of operating room work.

Personnel in the operating room can be divided into 4 main groups:

1. The surgeon and his medical assistants, who are professional physicians. They may include private physicians, family practitioners, and several levels of learners, such as the resident, the interne and the medical student.

2. The anesthesiologist and his assistants, who may be physicians and/or nurses. In large hospitals the department of anestheia may be directed by a physician and several associates, as well as learners. As part of the team and even directing some departments are nurse anesthetists. These are professional nurses who have taken additional qualifying work in the field of anesthesiology.

3. The operating room supervisor and her staff of nursing personnel. This group can be divided into professional and nonprofessional workers. Professional nurses are licensed graduate nurses, and they hold the positions of assistant supervisor, head nurses and staff nurses. Professional nurses are directly responsible for the teaching, the supervision and the guidance of nonprofessional workers.

The operating room supervisor is the administrative head of the operating room and as such is responsible for leadership and the coordination of all activities in the operating room. She may be directly responsible to the director of nursing, the hospital administrator or the chief surgeon.

Another segment of professional nursing is headed by an operating room clinical instructor, who is directly responsible for the teaching and the supervision of professional nursing students (but only if the hospital is used by a school of nursing). If there is no school of nursing, there may be a professional nurse in charge of in-service education.

Nonprofessional or auxiliary personnel in the operating room include the licensed practical nurse, the surgical technical aide, the nurse's aide and/or maid, the orderly, the porter and the secretary. These individuals are directly responsible to the professional nursing staff.

A surgical technical aide is a selected lay person who, through a well-planned and well-organized course of instruction, is prepared to function intelligently under the direct and continuous supervision of qualified professional nurses within hospital areas intimately concerned with the principles and practices of surgical asepsis, i.e., operating room, delivery room, emergency room, and central service department.[1]

4. Housekeeping department. This division may be a part of the nursing department, or it may be a separate entity. At any rate, the function of personnel in this department is an obvious one: to keep the operating room clean.

Individuals who work in an operating room seem to possess certain common necessary qualities regardless of the position held. Each person must be *healthy,* both mentally and physically. He is *interested* in his work, and that is why he is there. He recognizes his role as a *team member,* and as such he abides by team rules, which include *respect, patience, tact* and *understanding.* At times these virtues may be tested when emergencies arise. Even so, his reaction is to be *calm* and *quick-thinking.* He soon learns that *planning* and *organization* are essential

[1] American Hospital Association: Surgical Technical Aide, Instructor's Manual, p. 5, Chicago, 1954.

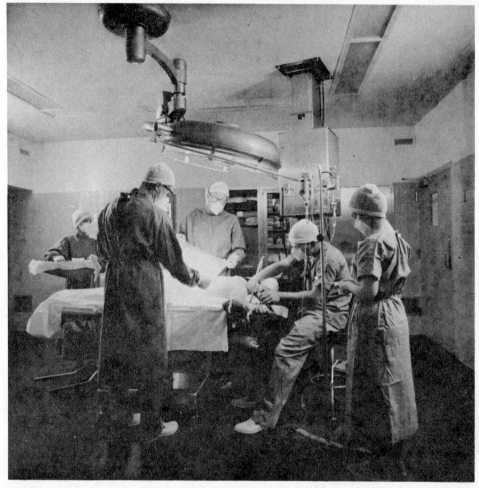

Fig. 2. The operating room of today.

to proper functioning. With good planning and foresight he is able *to anticipate* the needs of the patient, the surgeon and the anesthesiologist.

Every member of the operating team is a learner: *there is no end to learning!* This is accomplished by individual questions, conferences, in-service programs, reading, and the interest and initiative of the learner. A most valuable learning tool in the operating room is simply *to listen*. As a surgeon with his assistants scrubs for an operation, as he converses with the anesthesiologist, as he collaborates with the operating room supervisor, valuable information is offered which can help each assistant to understand better the immediate task ahead. Communication and close collaboration among the team leaders (surgeon, anesthesiologist and professional nurse) and the passing of information on to their associates are the keystone in the successful performance of a team.

Each assistant, student or aide must demonstrate the ability to perform designated tasks and *to follow directions* with or without supervision. This means that each worker must be *honest* and *trustworthy* in carrying out the various tasks assigned. Not to do so may jeopardize the life of a patient; for example, using an unsterile instrument can cause infection. Even the entire operating team could be adversely affected, as might occur if a woolen blanket were brought into the area where an explosive anesthetic gas is being used (friction of wool creates sparks that are capable of igniting a gas).

In the world of the operating room the work of every member of the team, from the surgeon who performs the operation to the important person who cleans the floor, is significant. If a worker is not conscientious and willing to do his assignment well, a patient may die. This is a high price to pay for carelessness, unconcern or even dishonesty. On the other hand, there are the great satisfactions of doing a job well, working with outstanding individuals, and observing the marvels of surgery as increasing numbers of persons are helped to live more productive lives.

OBJECTIVES OF A PROGRAM IN OPERATING ROOM TECHNOLOGY

These are:

1. To know the meaning of asepsis and to recognize the importance of one's own part in maintaining aseptic conditions in the operating room.

2. To offer the best team support to the patient, the surgeon, the anesthetist, and the professional nurse.

3. To be impressed with and have respect for the patient's right to privacy, dignity and safety; this implies that each team member be considerate, dependable and honest.

4. To develop habits of economy as they apply to time and the care and the preparation of supplies and equipment.

5. To gain satisfaction from doing a job well which is interesting, essential and soul-satisfying, because it is related to serving others.

6. To understand common operative procedures and their significance to the patient and his well-being.

7. To practice good personal health habits inasmuch as they affect patient care in the operating room.

8. To understand the value of records and reporting as well as the legal responsibility of each member of the operating team toward himself and the patient.

9. To be instilled with the· importance of observing lines of authority and to support all policies.

10. To understand the kinds of emergency that can develop in the operating room, and what one's particular role is in such an event.

Bibliography

Ginsberg, F.: Surgical technical aides help to solve a nursing shortage, Mod. Hosp. 96:102, June, 1961.

Gould, E. A.: The operating room nurse . . . is she a dying species?, A.O.R.N.J. 1:47–48, March–April 1963.

Owens, E. J.: From one O.R. nurse to another, Am. J. Nurs. 63:105–109, February 1963.

Peers, J. G.: Today's challenge to the professional operating room nurse, A.O.R.N.J. 1:69–73, January–February 1964.

Rockwell, V.: What is an OR nurse?, A.O.R.N.J. 1:10, January–February 1963.

Sister M. V. Clare: Breaking the OR Barrier, Am. J. Nurs. 64:116–118, September 1964.

CHAPTER 2

HOSPITAL AND OPERATING ROOM ORGANIZATION

TYPES OF HOSPITALS : HOSPITAL ORGANIZATION : OPERATING
ROOM ORGANIZATION

TYPES OF HOSPITALS

Hospitals are the 5th largest industry in this country. There are different kinds of hospitals, totaling over 7,000 in the United States, with various types of administrative organizations. To name some of them, there are:[1]

1. The voluntary, nonprofit hospital. This type of institution represents almost half the hospitals in the country. It is a corporation controlled by a group of selected trustees working without monetary compensation, who are charged with the moral, the ethical and the legal responsibility of administering the public funds which support the hospital. The Trustees can be held legally liable for the actions of everyone who works in the hospital from the director to the elevator boy.

If, at the end of a year, there is any excess of income over the expenses of the hospital, this excess is returned to the corporation and applied toward future deficits or building programs.

This agency serves the community in which it is located and strives constantly to improve the quality of patient care. Representatives of the total citizenry serve on the Board of Trustees.

2. Government hospitals. These may be either federal or state supported and controlled. Patients admitted to these institutions are entitled to the care they need and will receive. Examples of these are state psychiatric or tuberculosis

[1] Hospitals, guide issue of the American Hospital Association, August 1964.

11

hospitals, Veterans Administration hospitals or long-term general hospitals for senior citizens or rehabilitation. It may be necessary that employees take and pass civil service examinations before they can be employed. The employees usually are given more fringe benefits, such as retirement, higher salaries, etc., than those offered by the nonprofit, voluntary hospital. The administrative organization of these institutions can be similar to that of a corporation.

3. Proprietary, nonvoluntary hospitals. These are profit-making organizations controlled by one or more individuals. Profits are distributed by dividends to the owner or owners. The owner could be one individual physician, a partnership or a corporation. The administrator of such a hospital is not eligible for membership in the American College of Hospital Administrators, and few are accredited by the Joint Commission of Accreditation of Hospitals (JCAH), because minimum standards of the JCAH are most often not met. Before such a hospital can be opened, a state license is required. This is the only control the public has over the operation of a profit-making hospital.

HOSPITAL ORGANIZATION

The larger the institution, the more complex is its organization. However, whether it is large or small, each individual hospital must have a basic organizational plan for the performance of its functions. The operating room technologist, as well as all other personnel employed in the hospital, should know his or her relationship to other individuals and departments in the hospital. (Fig. 3)

AIMS OF THE HOSPITAL

The hospital exists for the promotion of the general health of society and derives its purposes from the needs of the community that it serves. The aims of an institution are reflected in the policies set up to govern its activities. The organization of the institution means the formal structure of authority that is to define, to distribute and to provide for the coordination of the tasks in their several contributions to the whole.

The Board of Trustees carries the weight of the complete function of the hospital and the achievement of its purposes, but it delegates authority to the Administrator or Director to enable him to organize, to plan, to direct and to coordinate the activities of hospital departments and services needed to achieve, within the budget available, the aims that have been set forth.

LINES OF AUTHORITY

The person in charge of each hospital department is responsible for the total function and performance of the employees in that department. With the authority invested in him by his immediate superior, he has the right to take such action and to require it of others as will enable him to accomplish the goals of the

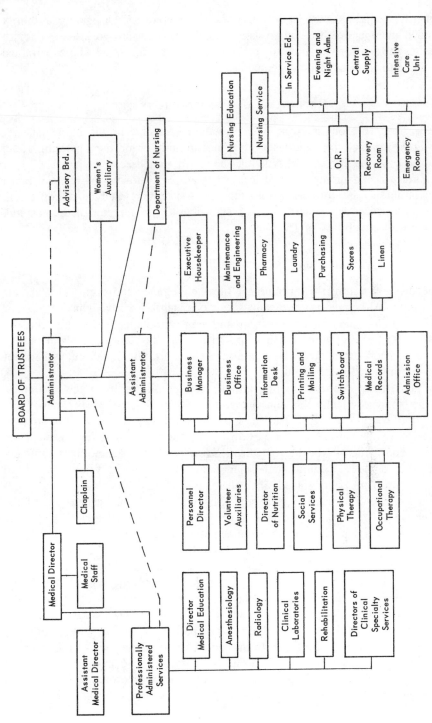

Fig. 3. Typical hospital organizational plan.

department. He administers and supervises the employees, delegating authority
to qualified members of his staff to assist him in the over-all work load. They in
turn assign the tasks to be done to other department employees who are trained
and qualified to carry out such assignments.

DELEGATION OF RESPONSIBILITY

The supervisor (person in charge) is directly responsible to his immediate superior. For example, the supervisor of a patient unit or of the operating room
is responsible to the Director of Nursing Service or the Director of Nursing.

The Director of Nursing could delegate her authority to one of her assistants,
but she ultimately is still responsible for her assistant as well as all others in
the Nursing Service Department. She is responsible to the Director of the hospital,
and he in turn to the Board of Trustees.

INTERDEPARTMENTAL RELATIONSHIPS

Each department within the structure of hospital organization is an integral part
of the whole. Although its particular specialty, such as x-ray, housekeeping or
nursing service, is its primary function and concern, its activities must be co-
ordinated with those of other departments to achieve the desired result in patient
care. Within each department there is also an organizational pattern with direct
lines of authority and responsibility.

How departments depend on one another can be shown by a few examples.
(1) If the laboratory technician complained to the pathologist that specimens from
the operating room were coming to the laboratory too late in the day for processing unless someone stayed overtime to do it, and the pathologist reprimanded the
operating room orderly who brought them down the next day, nothing construc-
tive would have been accomplished. In fact, ill feelings might well be generated
without the problem being solved. If, instead, the pathologist discussed the problem with the operating room supervisor (who may not have been aware of the
scheduled hours of work of the laboratory personnel), it is likely that her cooperation could solve the problem immediately and help to establish better
cooperation between the operating room and the laboratory. (2) The nursing
unit which prepares the patient for surgery is responsible for completed preparation as ordered by the doctor. If, when the patient arrives in surgery, it is found
that the preoperative medication has not been given, or that any other order left
by the physician has not been carried out, it could delay unnecessarily the scheduled surgery, and certainly it would upset the patient. (3) Everything could be
set up for a patient in surgery, sterile instruments and linens, but if, due to poor
housekeeping, the operating room were dusty or dirty, the patient after a successful
surgical repair could develop an infection from lack of environmental control of
the cleanliness of the operating room.

OPERATING ROOM ORGANIZATION

The department of surgery, which includes the operating room, is one of many departments within the hospital. The supervisor or director of the operating room may be directly responsible for the activities of the department to the Director of Nursing, the chief of surgery, or the Administrator of the hospital, depending on the organizational plan and the policies of the institution. In any event, the operating room supervisor is responsible for the planning and the administration of nursing service in the operating room and for the functioning of all nursing and auxiliary personnel in her department. (Fig. 4)

Personnel in the Operating Room

These include:

1. Surgeons. The surgeon is in complete charge of his operating team. He is a private practicing physician and surgeon, or he may be employed by the hospital for specific duties.

2. Resident physicians and internes. These physicians usually function in the role of the surgeon's assistants, learning as they gain experience. In some instances a resident physician may do a surgical procedure, and thereby he becomes the person in charge of the team at that time.

3. The anesthesiologist and his assistants may be physicians or specially trained nurses.

4. Nursing service personnel. Although nurses and other members of the nursing service department work very closely with the surgeon and his assistants, there still are distinct nursing responsibilities that do not directly affect the physician or his assistants except as they affect the care of the patients. For example, the physicians do not, as a rule, directly inspect or supervise the sterilization of instruments or supplies to be used in surgery. However, if there should be any indication that the procedure in use was inadequate, it would be of deep concern to all physicians. The personnel in the operating room work within the framework of hospital, administrative and operating room policies.

The entire functioning of the nursing service organization is the responsibility of the operating room supervisor. She coordinates the activities of her department with other departments in the hospital and with her own employees and the surgeons. She participates in policy making, infection control committee activities, operating room nursing committee, in-service education, preparation and writing of procedures and job descriptions; and she delegates authority and responsibility to members of her staff. Each team member must know what his task or assignment is and how to accomplish it. If an assignment is made that is confusing, or if the worker has not been properly instructed, he must make this known to the person to whom he is responsible. The lack of such communication, or a small mistake, could cost the life of a patient. Auxiliary personnel in the operating

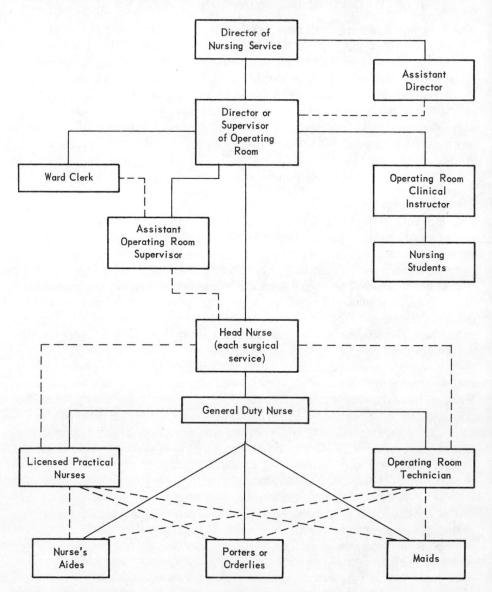

Fig. 4. Operating room organizational chart. A typical organizational plan for the operating room in a nonprofit, voluntary hospital is shown. The solid lines indicate direct lines of authority and responsibility. Authority is shown from the top of the chart downward, and the same lines show responsibility upward. The broken lines indicate a cooperative relationship and channels of communication between workers.

room are selected after careful screening. Not everyone is suited to work in this vital area of patient care. The demands of service in surgery are inspiring and elating to some, giving great personal satisfaction from the service rendered to the patient, but the work may be frightening and depressing to others.

The auxiliary personnel in the operating room work under the direct supervision of the general staff nurse. She in turn is directly responsible to the head nurse of the surgery service to which she is assigned. The head nurse is responsible to the supervisor or her assistant.

The nursing service personnel act as team members to provide the best possible service and facilities to the patient undergoing surgery. This includes not only the practice of aseptic technics but maintaining a safe environment, meeting the psychological and physical needs of the patient, keeping records, and preserving her own physical fitness, as well as assisting the surgeons and their assistants.

Responsibility to the patient is an important aspect of operating room nursing service. There are also the responsibilities that team members have to one another, to themselves, to the patient's family and to the community at large. With all members of the team working together conscientiously, the patient is given the best chance of recovery.

Delegation of Responsibility. Each secretary, maid, orderly, nurse's aide, licensed practical nurse, nurse's assistant, and operating room technologist, as well as the graduate nurse, has individual and coordinating responsibilities with all other members of the team in the common cause of furnishing the quality of patient care desirable. Job descriptions are mandatory so that each person knows what is expected of him, and to whom he is responsible.

Moral and Ethical Responsibility. Conformity to accepted standards of conduct, honesty, consideration of others, and observation of policies and rules and regulations must be practiced by all personnel at all times. The constant aim of optimum patient care must be the primary objective in the minds and actions of all members of the team. Only conscientious performance of the job at hand is acceptable.

Operating room personnel frequently come in contact with the friends and families of patients and are prepared to be considerate and courteous, regardless of the situation. For example, a patient admitted to the outpatient department with severe injuries may be taken directly to the operating room for surgery. Operating room personnel may be dispatched to transport the patient from one department to the other. If the patient is seriously hurt, and the family desires to have a spiritual adviser present, the situation must be handled with tact and understanding. The patient cannot be allowed to bleed to death while he is waiting, if there is a delay, and yet the wishes of the patient and/or his family cannot be ignored. Either the physician or the nurse should handle this kind of situation because of their greater experience and preparation. The nurse's assistant or orderly (as the case may be) should not attempt to make the decisions needed at that moment.

Poise and the use of good common sense in all situations charged with emotional overtones are requisites for operating room workers. Since people are human, occasions could arise in which tension and anxiety are present. It is then the responsibility of other team members to keep calm, to try to heal the breach as quickly as possible, and to proceed with the job at hand. Operating room policies must be followed. This, too, is a moral responsibility of every worker in the operating room.

Legal Responsibility. Although the supervisor is responsible for the entire functioning of her department and all members of her staff, each member of the staff in turn is responsible for his or her individual actions. (See Chap. 13.)

Communications. If the team is to work smoothly and effectively, many types of communication will be used by the various members. Verbal orders must be clear, not mumbled. At times this becomes a problem because of the various tones of voices, and with a face mask in place, some voices sound less clear or audible. If there is any doubt as to what has been said, a request for repetition of the instruction is in order.

When a team has been working together, a spirit of comradery develops, a "feeling," a mutual understanding most difficult to define. Many times the scrub assistant and the circulating nurse may communicate with each other solely by hand signals, the eyebrows or eye expressions. These signs might not be meaningful to others, but team members who have worked together well can interpret them with no difficulty.

An alert circulating nurse, seeing beads of perspiration on the surgeon's forehead, prepares to remove them with a towel, standing by until an appropriate time is indicated; actually she may not say anything to the surgeon. He in turn expects this help and usually does not need to ask someone to wipe his brow.

The handling of a human body is another form of communication. It makes a great deal of difference to a patient whether he is treated gently with due regard for his personal dignity and pain or handled roughly, without feeling, like an inanimate object to be moved from one place to another. Each worker and each patient is an individual with personal worth and dignity, and he should be respected and treated as such.

Because of the element of human individuality, personalities also differ. No hard and fast rules can be applied to fit the care of *every* patient coming to the operating room, but experience teaches one how to relate to each patient. In other words, one would not attempt to tell an anecdote to a drowsy, sedated patient any more than he would attempt to confide his personal problems to a crying child.

Telephone calls to the operating room should be kept at a minimum. It is true that many calls are necessary, but all personal and unnecessary calls should be prohibited. It is best to have a department secretary or ward clerk at one location to take incoming calls and to relay necessary messages. Except in an emergency, interrupting members of the surgical team when they are operating is an unwise practice.

Any written communications between the operating room and other hospital departments, or vice versa, must be legible and precise. (See Chap. 9.) Forms used for requisitions or records must be filled out accurately and properly signed, depending on the policies of the hospital and the operating room.

Noise interrupts communication. It is distracting and undesirable for both the patients and the conscientious people who are members of the surgical team. Every effort should be made, in keeping with the accomplishment of the task at hand, to reduce noise to a minimum. Unnecessary banging of metal basins or instruments, loud voices or laughter, the slamming of doors or audible conversations should be eliminated. There is a time and a place for expression of lightheartedness, but it does not belong in surgery when a patient is on the table.

ORGANIZATION OF AREAS IN THE OPERATING ROOM

Patient Areas (Fig. 5). The physical plan of the operating room will vary from one institution to another just as the organizational plan may differ. However, there generally are basic components in most.

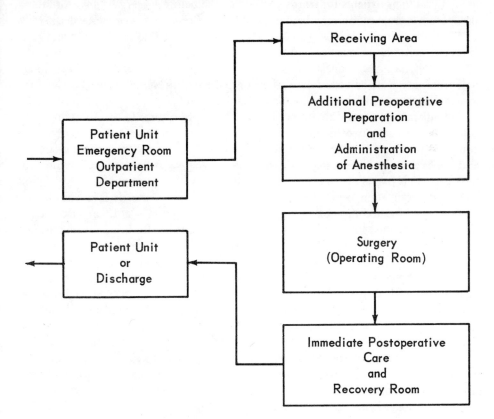

Fig. 5. Patient areas.

Beyond the point of the patient-receiving area, the operating room is considered to be a restricted area, and unauthorized personnel are not permitted.

Personnel are allowed beyond the dressing rooms only when they are properly attired in conductive shoes or overshoes and scrub clothes. This area is totally restricted except for operating room personnel, authorized persons, and patients. This rule must be enforced rigidly for the safety of the patients and the personnel. First, it involves bacteriologic safety. Bacteria may be dispersed from clothes and shoes that have been worn elsewhere. Second, there is an explosive hazard. All personnel and equipment must be properly grounded—personnel by the wearing of special shoes—when combustible anesthetic gases are used in the operating room.

The patient comes to surgery from the patient unit, the emergency room or the outpatient department, depending on the nature of his surgical treatment and condition. From any of these three admission places he is received in the operating room in a specific receiving area where the operating room nurse takes over his care. He should not be left alone in a sedated state; nor should he feel abandoned at this crucial time and place. There must be someone with him who can give the moral support and the supervision that his condition requires. Surgeons also are able to visit their patients for words or reassurance before surgery begins. Additional preoperative preparation may be completed in the receiving area as needed.

After the surgery is completed, the patient is taken to an immediate post-operative care unit or recovery room, where he is kept until his condition, evaluated by the physician or the anesthesiologist, indicates that he is ready to return to the unit from which he came. In case of an outpatient with minor surgery under local anesthesia, the patient may be discharged to his home.

Outpatients (patients who are not hospitalized) often come to the operating room suite for cystoscopic examinations, done in a "cysto" room that is especially equipped for this procedure. Facilities are provided there for the patient's comfort and needs without interfering with surgery in progress or violating the rules and the restrictions that apply to people coming into the surgical suite.

A cast room often is provided in the operating room suite. It is advisable that this room be located in another hospital area; but when it is not, care is taken to prevent plaster dust from entering other parts of the suite. Both inpatients and outpatients may have casts applied. Facilities for receiving both types of patients should be provided.

In many hospitals a quiet, cheerful room located outside the operating suite or nearby is furnished for the families of patients who are in surgery. Although isolated from the bustle of a busy unit, they are near the operating room, conveniently located where the surgeon or the nurses can keep them informed of the condition of the patient in surgery.

Operating Room Personnel Areas. The operating room suite contains the work areas necessary for the personnel to carry out their respective activities. The areas allocated are dependent on the size and the type of the hospital and the volume and the types of surgical procedures performed. (See Fig. 6.)

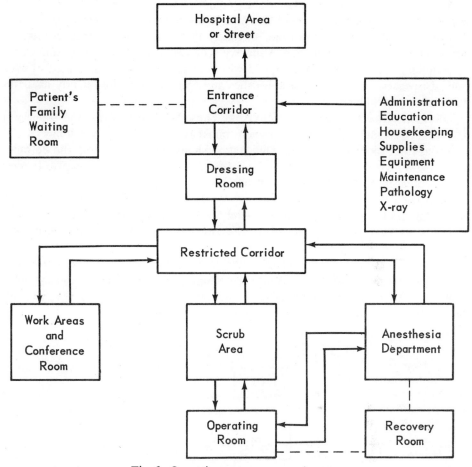

Fig. 6. Operating room personnel areas.

The coordinated activities of other hospital departments are arranged as necessary through the supervisor (or the person in charge) according to the policies that have been developed.

Dressing rooms and lounges are provided. Street clothes or hospital uniforms are changed in the dressing room for operating room attire. The person then is ready to work in the restricted area of the operating room.

Dressing rooms include showers, lavatory, toilets, mirrors, locker space adequate for each employee for street clothes and shoes, and extra lockers for visiting surgeons. Laundry hampers are provided for soiled surgical garb, and cabinets or drawers for freshly laundered scrub clothes in quantities adequate for the needs of the staff. A lounge may be shared by all personnel for coffee breaks, or these facilities may be set up in conjunction with the two dressing rooms.

Scrub Room. The scrub sinks, usually equipped with foot or knee hot and cold water controls, or elbow controls, are in a room adjoining the operating room. It is here that the surgeons and other members of the team scrub their hands and arms before gowning and gloving in surgery. The containers for the antiseptics used in scrubbing technic also are equipped with foot controls and are located at each sink. Dispensers containing sterile brushes and nail files are conveniently available to the person scrubbing.

Offices. OPERATING ROOM SUPERVISOR. The office provided for the supervisor includes a desk and a chair, filing cabinets, bookcase and communication media.

SECRETARY OR WARD CLERK. This station should be located near the entrance of the suite, where all personnel and patients entering can be seen easily. It most often is adjacent to the operating room supervisor's office.

ANESTHESIA OFFICE. This space may or may not be in the operating suite, depending on the volume and the scope of the work of the anesthesia department. An anesthesia workroom is needed for the care and the maintenance of equipment and supplies.

Conference Rooms. A conference room should be provided for staff and in-service education meetings and for the student teaching program. It should be equipped with appropriate teaching materials, blackboard, projector and screen, large table with chairs, and other needed equipment and teaching aids.

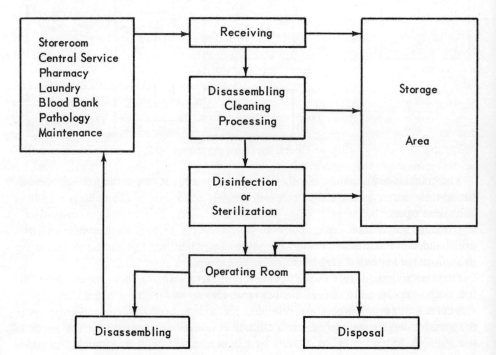

Fig. 7. Supplies and equipment areas.

Supplies and Equipment Area (Fig. 7). Supplies and equipment are requisitioned from the department that issues them (drugs from the pharmacy, sponges and sutures from the storeroom, sterile packs from central service, etc.). They are received at a central place in the operating suite, usually at the ward secretary's station, and from there are stored for future use, processed for use or sterile storage, or used immediately. Supplies and instruments that have been used in surgery are disassembled, cleaned and reprocessed in a clean-up area, although some hospitals take care of these tasks in central service. Equipment or supplies from other departments that have been used in surgery are cleaned and returned to the place of origin. Waste materials are discarded in appropriate receptacles. The utilization of available space for the storage of sterile and unsterile supplies is the decision of the supervisor.

Sterilizing Room. This room contains instrument washer-sterilizers, ultrasonic cleaning units, a clean-up area, a solutions warmer, and possibly a large standard autoclave and a high speed sterilizer. Between the two major surgery rooms in some operating room suites is a substerilizing room equipped with a high speed and instrument washer-sterilizer. A flushing rim hopper sink often is located in this area.

Supply and Storage Rooms. GENERAL STORAGE ROOM (UNSTERILE EQUIPMENT). There are numerous miscellaneous materials that need a storage place when they are not in use. Large equipment, such as a portable x-ray machine, an electrosurgical unit or a cast cart, extra I.V. poles, spare parts for operating tables, carriers for transporting gas cylinders, and portable operating room lights, as well as other equipment, clutters the operating room or the corridor when not in use. This equipment should be kept in a general storage room. The size of the room would be determined by the amount of equipment to be stored, which in turn would be dependent on the size of the operating room suite and the volume and the kinds of surgery done.

UNSTERILE SUPPLIES. The unsterile linens used on operating room tables and stretchers, armboard covers, etc., usually are kept in a corridor closet near the operating room door or on a shelf inside the room. The quantity used of this kind of linen is minimal in comparison with that used in a patient unit.

Many instruments used infrequently may be stored in an instrument cabinet, where they are clean but unsterile. For example, delicate eye instruments are stored in special plastic boxes so that they will not be damaged. In some hospitals such instruments are cleaned, sterilized and stored for future use. Instrument storage is organized, those instruments used for specific types of surgery being in one section of an instrument cabinet and those for other types in another.

Orthopedic pins, screws, etc., usually are selected according to the needs of the individual case because of the many sizes and types available.

STERILE SUPPLY CLOSET. Two factors that influence the size and the design of the sterile storage room are the way in which the supplies are stored and the quantity needed for daily use and reserve. Sterile supplies, except those in the operating room on shelves, are centralized and arranged in this room so that they are readily accessible and easily checked for replacement. The sterile shelves are filled directly from the autoclave racks after the cooling process is completed, or the supply is replenished after the central service delivery. For easy identification the storage area is divided; linen packs, instrument sets, gloves, basins and trays are kept separate.

SOLUTIONS: DRUGS, BLOOD. Flasks of solutions for use in the operating room (sterile saline and distilled water) and intravenous solutions* usually are kept in a separate closet or room. The solution-warmer cabinet is refilled from this supply as needed. Solutions used for refilling transfer forceps containers and for chemical disinfection in general are dispensed usually to the operating room in gallon containers. There must be a convenient place to keep these large bottles or containers. Unsterile solutions should be stored apart from sterile solutions. A refrigerator is essential for the storing of blood and some drugs.

Porter's Clean-up Room (Janitor's Closet). An ideal plan is to have a closet in each substerilizing room between two operating rooms to store the equipment needed for cleaning the adjacent rooms.

When one closet is used, it accommodates all supplies and equipment for cleaning rooms after each operation, and its most suitable location is a centralized area of the suite. Wet objects, such as cleaning cloths or mop heads, should be sent to the laundry with the linen after each operation. Mops, bucket and wringer or vacuuming equipment should be located here. Detergents and cleaning solutions should be stored here on shelves. The room should be equipped with an exhaust ventilating system so that the discharged air and odors do not enter other areas of the suite.

Most hospitals have incinerators for the disposal of wastes and contaminated materials. There may be a special container in this room for these items, although in some hospitals wastes are collected in a container in the clean-up area.

Workroom. In this room, usually located in an area remote from the actual operating rooms, unsterile linens are folded, and packs and other materials are assembled and prepared for autoclaving. The Central Service has taken over the responsibility of this function in many institutions, although many surgeries still process their linen in the workroom despite bacteriologic hazards. The workroom usually is staffed by trained nursing aides under the supervision of a professional nurse.

Dark Room. X-ray pictures taken in the operating room are developed in the dark room by x-ray personnel who service and maintain its equipment. The purpose of having an x-ray unit in the operating room is to enable the surgeon to check the work that he is doing, to see the x-ray pictures quickly even though they still are wet, and then to resume the surgery.

Linking Areas. *Corridor.* The entrance corridor should be equipped with mechanically operated double doors to allow for safe passage of patient stretchers into and out of the operating room suite. The part of the corridor up to the ward clerk's desk

* Also sterile suture jars if they still are used.

is considered to be an unrestricted area and/or a receiving area for patients in many institutions in which there is no other available space. If there is no space for a specific receiving area, stretchers and beds of patients in surgery must be stored somewhere while surgery is in progress. The corridor may be used for this purpose, although there is general agreement that provision for a receiving or waiting area for patients is a more desirable arrangement.

The usual 8-foot-wide corridor may be inadequate if it serves these other functions as well as its normal one of permitting flow of traffic and equipment between the various surgery units. If it is not cluttered and crowded, a width of 8 feet is adequate, provided that doors do not open into it. The corridor must conform to local codes in respect to width, egress, ingress, fire exits, etc.

Placing a conductivity meter (see Chap. 7) in the corridor between the dressing rooms and the restricted area is the best location for reminding personnel leaving the dressing rooms to check the conductivity of their shoes before entering any hazardous area. Preferably, this machine is recessed so that the metal plates do not protrude and interfere with corridor traffic.

A bulletin board near the ward clerk's desk is useful for posting operating room schedules and personnel time sheets and assignments. Other informative and educational materials placed on the board should be arranged attractively and changed frequently to keep reader interest.

Elevator. An elevator may be used for surgery patients only, in which case its doors open directly into the unrestricted corridor of the operating room; or patients may need to share a bank of elevators that are used by other hospital traffic and personnel. In this event the interest of the patients is best served by having the elevators located as near to the entrance corridor of the suite as possible. Air conditioning is needed in elevators to assist in temperature control and elimination of odors. During peak surgery hours patients should be transported in elevators that do not have visitors and other hospital personnel and equipment riding with them. With planning it is possible to set aside the number of elevators needed for surgical patients without inconveniencing others.

REVIEW QUESTIONS:
1. What purpose does a hospital organizational plan serve? Is this important to patient care? If so, how?
2. What are some of the basic differences in hospital administrative organizations?
3. Explain what is meant by "interdepartmental relationships."
4. Draw a representation of your operating room organizational plan, placing names of your co-workers with their work titles in the appropriate places.
5. What information should a "job description" contain?
6. In what ways do we communicate with other people? Name some of the factors which influence the effectiveness or the failure to communicate.
7. What are some of the factors that influence the size and the design of storage areas?

Bibliography

Gifford, D. L.: Basic Planning of the Operating Room Suite, reprint from Hospital Topics, May 1963.

Hospitals, guide issue of the American Hospital Association, August 1964.

Safe Practice for Hospital Operating Rooms, Bulletin No. 56, National Fire Protection Association, 1962.

Smith, Warwick: Planning the Surgical Suite, New York, F. W. Dodge Corp., 1960.

UNIT 2

*Principles and Practices
of Surgical Asepsis*

CHAPTER 3

ESSENTIALS OF MICROBIOLOGY

INTRODUCTION : CLASSIFICATION OF MICROORGANISMS :

BACTERIA : FUNGI : VIRUSES : BODY DEFENSES

INTRODUCTION

The science of microbiology is a fascinating and exciting one, providing, as it does, some answers to many remarkable questions about our life. Basically, it is a field in which you have some background of knowledge. Why from the days of your early childhood were you taught to wash your hands carefully before eating, to practice good personal hygiene, to wash and dry clothes and dishes, to refrigerate pasteurized milk, to take vaccines and other injections? You did all this and much more "to kill germs." What are germs? They are living creatures, as alive as plants and animals that you see. Everywhere on earth there are fantastic numbers of tiny living creatures that are too small to be seen with the naked eye, and therefore we usually are not conscious of their presence. If we wish to see them, we use a microscope. Some of these creatures are so minute that a special electron microscope must be used. A more appropriate term for "germ" is microbe or microorganism. The microbes of greatest concern to us are that group called the *bacteria* (a single organism of this group is a *bacterium*).

Your reference to "germs" was usually in relation to those bacteria which are *pathogenic*—that is, produce disease. Not *all* bacteria are pathogenic by any means. The vast majority of microorganisms are harmless (nonpathogenic) and have no connection with disease. Many bacteria are very useful to man. For instance, there are those in the intestinal tract that synthesize (help to produce) vitamin K, which is absorbed by the liver and used to control bleeding; other intestinal bacteria manufacture folic acid, a vitamin which prevents anemias.

Dairymen, agriculturists, leather tanners, food processors and many manufacturers are interested in certain kinds of microbes for practical reasons. Hospital personnel who devote themselves to the care of the sick also are concerned with a variety of bacterial forms. Many diseases are caused by the spread of bacteria and other types of microbes. The technic which forms a part of the routine care of patients is designed to destroy, to exclude or to avoid bacteria that may be harmful. Such technic is called *aseptic* (a = without; septic = infection). Keeping bacteria out of wounds during surgery and deliveries and out of emergency or dressing rooms can be accomplished safely by persons who clearly understand how to exclude and to destroy microorganisms.

CLASSIFICATION OF MICROORGANISMS

Microbiology is one branch of the greater science of biology, which includes studies of the nature of all living matter. Microbiology is a practical subject concerned with microscopic organisms, their form, structure, mode of life, and what they do particularly to human beings.

SEVEN MAIN GROUPS

Microorganisms may be found in seven main groups, which are listed as follows, with examples:
1. Algae—green plants. Pond scum. There are no known pathogenic forms.
2. Protozoa—microscopic animals. Amebae. They cause diseases such as malaria and amebic dysentery.
3. Yeasts—microscopic fungi. Bakers' yeast. They can cause diseases of the skin and other structures.
4. Molds—microscopic fungi. Woolly growth on damp bread. They can cause diseases, such as athlete's foot.
5. Bacteria—microscopic fungi. They cause diseases such as tuberculosis, dysentery, various "strep" and "staph" infections.
6. Rickettsiae—probably vegetable kingdom. They cause diseases like Rocky Mountain spotted fever.
7. Viruses. They cause diseases such as poliomyelitis, influenza, measles and the common cold.
Of the above forms bacteria and viruses are the most important for our purposes.

RELATIONSHIP BETWEEN MAN AND BACTERIA

There are three types of association among organisms:
1. **Symbiosis** (living together). In this relationship two kinds of organisms live together with mutual benefit. An example is the relationship between man and bacteria in the colon (large bowel). With constant temperature, food and darkness, bacteria live on fecal content, not human tissue. In return, the bacteria produce vitamin K and folic acid.
2. **Commensalism.** One kind of organism obtains its food from the host and thereby is benefited. The host is neither benefited nor harmed. An example is the

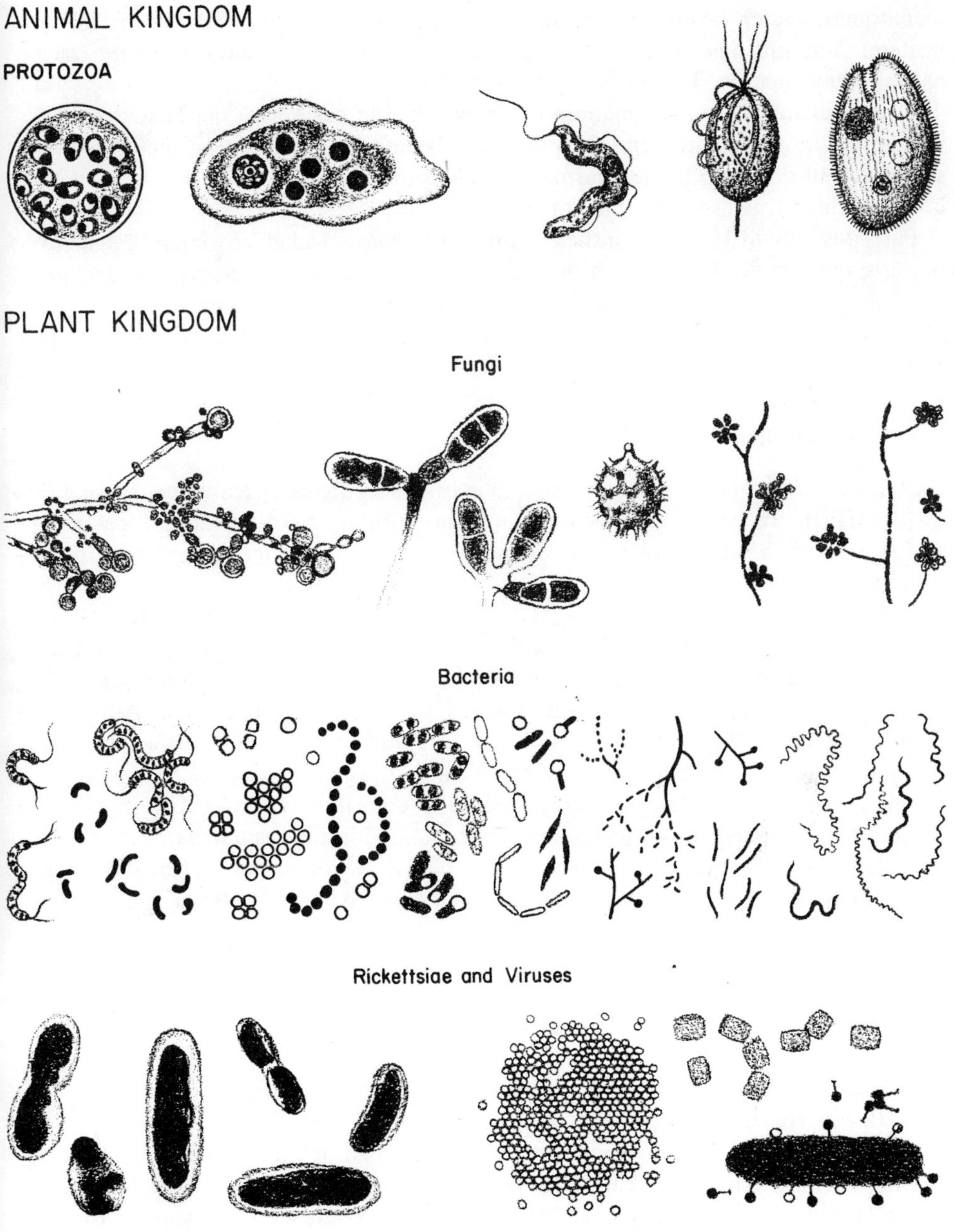

ANIMAL KINGDOM

PROTOZOA

PLANT KINGDOM

Fungi

Bacteria

Rickettsiae and Viruses

Fig. 8. Representative types of microorganisms. Not drawn to scale. (Von Gremp, Z., and Broadwell, L.: Practical Nursing: Study Guide and Review, ed. 2, Fig. 9, p. 50, Philadelphia, Lippincott, 1965)

commensal relationship between man and bacteria on the skin and the mucous membranes. Outer layers of skin are made up of dead cells and harbor many bacteria. The mucous membrane of the mouth, the nose and the alimentary tract harbor many bacteria. These are called normal flora.

3. **Parasitism.** This is a relationship in which one organism, the host, may be injured by the association, and the parasite is benefited. In parasitism the organism sustains itself on *living* tissue. Harmful parasites that cause disease are the result of invading microorganisms that infect the host.

Parasites should be distinguished from *saprophytes,* which are microorganisms that live only on dead tissue. Saprophytes are responsible for the decay, the decomposition and the disposition of dead animals, dead trees or plants, and refuse. Most of the saprophytes are harmless to man, although a few species can cause serious or fatal disease.

BACTERIA

Bacteria are microscopic plants which may measure in diameter from about 1/2500 to 1/500 inch. To give a more meaningful picture of the size of bacteria, it has been said that a drop of milk may contain as many as 100 million bacteria, and a particle the size of a pinhead, 8 million.

Unlike familiar plants, bacteria have no green coloring matter, roots, stems, leaves or flowers. Many bacteria may live for years without sunlight, air, food or water. Like all other living things, including ourselves, bacteria are made up of a substance called *protoplasm* (proto = primitive; plasm = substance). Although an exact definition has not been found, it is felt that protoplasm is a substance in which there occurs all of the complex chemical and physical reactions that produce life. It is usually transparent, watery, generally colorless and resembles raw egg white. The protoplasm of all living things is contained in tiny chambers or sacs that are called *cells.* Bacteria belong to the group of one-cell organisms. Their life work consists of feeding, excreting waste products and multiplying. (Fig. 9)

THE NATURE OF BACTERIA

Bacterial Forms. Bacteria may be classified according to shape in three main classes:

1. Cocci (coccus is the singular), round or ball-shaped organisms.
2. Bacilli (bacillus is the singular), rod or cigarette-shaped organisms.
3. Spirilla (spirillum is the singular), comma-shaped or spiral organisms.

Unlike the others, spirilla can move by themselves because of the long filaments which provide a wavy, whiplike motion like that of a tail. Our study primarily is concerned with cocci and bacilli.

Bacterial Structure. The protoplasmic mass (bacterial cell), whether it is a coccus or a bacillus, is composed of at least three special parts. First, to retain and to protect the jellylike internal substance and to give the cell form, there is a *cell wall* or *membrane* which is extremely thin. Food materials can pass through it, and waste materials out of it. The second portion, the gelatinous mass inside the cell wall, is *cytoplasm* (cyto = cell; plasm = substance). This may contain water droplets, food particles, pigment granules, and specialized protoplasm related to digestion and reproduction. It is here that the work of the cell is carried out. The third part of the cell, a very important structure without which the cell would die, is the *nucleus*. Unlike animal cells, in which definite globules condense near the center, bacterial cells are believed to have nuclei that are dispersed throughout the cytoplasm in the form of tiny granules.

Surrounding many species of bacteria is a *slime layer* or gelatinous envelope which is called a *capsule*. Because capsules seem to protect organisms from the usual bactericidal factors in body fluids, it is believed that capsules contribute to the *virulence* (disease-producing power) of the organisms. Therefore, encapsulation is peculiar to most pathogenic strains.

Bacterial Nutrition. Since these minute creatures have no mouths or teeth with which to eat, substances used as food must be in solution, as in other plants. The food soaks into the bacterium through the cell wall. The passage of fluids and dissolved materials through a thin membrane is called *osmosis*. Dissolved waste products pass outward through the cell wall by osmosis. Strangely enough, only the "right" substances pass into the cell for the absorption of food through the semipermeable membrane, and only waste products pass outward.

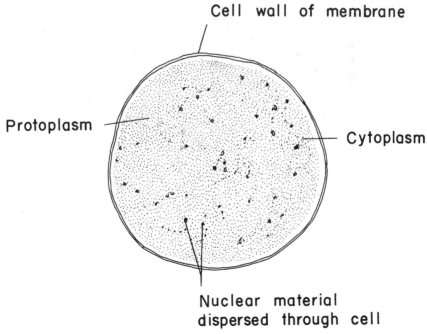

Fig. 9. Typical bacterial cell (coccus).

Bacterial Waste Products. In addition to harmless waste products, some species of bacteria give off various gases, whereas others provide enzymes or enzymelike substances. An enzyme is a chemical substance produced by a living cell. These chemicals in minute amounts cause remarkable changes to take place within the host. For instance, some bacterial cells provide enzymes which catalyze (speed up) our digestive processes. However, some enzymes or enzymelike substances produced by bacteria are toxic—that is, poisonous—and produce disease. Diphtheria toxin is one example.

Bacterial Growth. The following factors are important in the growth of bacteria:

1. *Moisture.* This is essential, since certain nutrient substances dissolve in the surrounding water and in this form can pass through the cell wall. Dehydration is used widely in preserving food, i.e., soups, eggs, potatoes, fruits and meats, since bacteria cannot multiply in the absence of water. However, drying does not kill all bacteria, although some are extremely sensitive in this respect. Some pathogenic bacteria may survive for long periods in dried pus, sputum, mucus or feces.

2. *Food.* The nature of the food demanded by bacteria varies with the species. Like the higher forms of life, bacteria need such chemical substances as oxygen, nitrogen, phosphorus and sulphur. Since bacteria have no roots, they must be suspended in solutions of food, where through osmosis their needs are met. Unlike the higher forms of plant life, their energy is obtained by complex chemical processes rather than from the sun's rays, which might injure them.

3. *Temperature.* Although food and water must be present, the temperature must be favorable for the particular strain. Organisms do not grow at uniform temperatures. Some, like those adapted to growth on the human body, flourish at 37° C. (98.6° F.). A few species on the bottom of the sea grow best at near-freezing temperatures 4–10° C. (39–50° F.). Refrigeration is used in homes, because we know that low temperatures will prevent the growth of many kinds of bacteria that cause souring or rancidity. However, low temperatures are seldom fatal to bacteria; some may remain viable (living) in a frozen state for years.

Some bacterial forms grow only at high temperatures ranging from 45–75° C. (113–177° F.), which is the temperature of water hot enough to produce scalding. Temperatures of 70° C. (158° F.) or higher will kill the actively growing *vegetative* forms of all except the thermophilic (heat-loving) bacteria. Some species which produce *spores* (these have coverings like tiny suits of armor) are most resistant and may live through boiling water, 100° C. (212° F.) and even higher temperatures for hours. The spore-forming bacteria are extremely dangerous. Sterilization technics designed to combat bacteria by means of heat will be discussed in the following chapter.

4. *Oxygen.* Some microorganisms grow only in the presence of free oxygen in the atmosphere. These forms are called *aerobes.* Some examples of aerobes are *Hemophilus influenzae,* a common parasite in man's nose and throat. This bacillus (rod) is not always present in the disease known as influenza, but it may be the cause of severe throat infections in children, meningitis or endocarditis. Another

Fig. 10. Reproductive phase of typical bacterial cell.

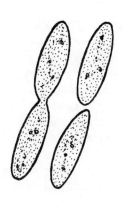

aerobe is *Pasteurella pestis,* the cause of bubonic plague. This bacillus carries a high mortality (death) rate. It is primarily a disease of rodents and is transmitted to man by infected fleas.

Anaerobes are those organisms that grow best in soil, swamp muck, bowel and other places where air cannot penetrate. The oxygen needed for their growth is obtained by decomposing chemical compounds that contain this element. One example of an anaerobe is *Clostridium perfringens,* the cause of gas gangrene, which often accompanies war wounds. Following tissue injury, the organism rapidly invades surrounding tissue, destroying it and producing marked gas formation. Another anaerobe is *Clostridium tetani,* the cause of tetanus or lockjaw. Tetanus spores may be swallowed without producing symptoms in man. However, when introduced into deep tissue structures through the skin on a dirty knife, a nail or a bayonet, they may invade, multiply and produce toxins which injure or kill tissue cells and paralyze body defenses.

Facultative bacteria, a very large group, are those which have the ability to adapt to an aerobic or an anaerobic environment. In other words, they can grow with free oxygen or without it. Examples are *Salmonella typhosa,* the cause of typhoid fever. This is a disease transmitted by water, milk, food or flies, causing acute generalized infection. *Micrococcus pyogenes (Staphylococcus),* a cause of boils and carbuncles, is another facultative organism. These bacteria can enter the broken and the unbroken skin to produce infection, causing pus. Strict aseptic technic in surgery can reduce the possibility of staphylococcal and other infections.

5. *Acidity and Alkalinity.* Many bacteria, particularly the pathogens, are destroyed or prevented from growing by making slight variations in their fluid environment. Pickled foods will "keep" indefinitely without refrigeration because the high acid content will prevent bacterial growth. For this reason it is well to know the acid-alkaline relationship of the various chemicals to be considered for the purposes of disinfection. (See Chap. 4.)

These factors and others provide a framework of understanding on which to base procedures that control bacterial reproduction.

Bacterial Reproduction. The multiplication of bacteria is considered to be asexual; that is, it is generally believed that no fertilization is needed, and that the cells are without sex. When the conditions for the growth of a particular species exist, and when the maximum size of each cell has been reached, the cell splits across the short axis to form two new cells. If the conditions still are favorable, the cells grow to their maximum size and split again. This simple reproductive cycle takes place for *most* bacterial cells.

The rate of cell division of bacterial forms is far more rapid than that in higher forms of life, although it varies with the species and with the conditions affecting the growth of the organisms. Some divide slowly, but most of them reproduce rapidly, every 20 to 30 minutes in the active phase when all conditions are ideal. However, as soon as the available food and water decrease, and waste products accumulate, cell division becomes slower until reproduction ceases. Certain drugs and chemicals can cause the slowdown or the cessation of cell division. If the chemical causes cessation of cell division, and the organisms die, the chemical is said to be *bactericidal*. If the chemical stops reproduction but does not kill the organisms, it is said to be *bacteriostatic*.

Cell Grouping. As was stated earlier, the bacterial forms of interest to us are *cocci* (spheres) and *bacilli* (rods). Among the cocci, and to a lesser extent the bacilli and the spirilla, the growing cells tend to form characteristic groupings that help in laboratory recognition of species. Most of the common cocci occur in groups of two or more cells. Cocci in pairs are called *diplococci*. These may cause meningitis and pneumonia. Those which form chains are called *streptococci*. Although many strains are harmless, these organisms may cause endocarditis, scarlet fever, tonsillitis, etc. Irregular masses resembling clusters of grapes are called *staphylococci*. These are the most prevalent organisms on the human body; they are present on the human skin and usually are harmless. Some strains may cause boils, carbuncles, stitch abscesses, pneumonia, etc.

Bacilli like cocci show marked variation in their basic shape. Although rod-shaped, some are short, thick and straight, whereas others are long, slender and curved. They are widely distributed, and many species are known to be very helpful to man. Döderlein's bacillus, which maintains the acidity of vaginal secretions, is extremely helpful in preventing infection. *Escherichia coli* (colon bacillus), which constitutes about 75 per cent of the living bacteria in feces, and other aerobic and anaerobic bacilli under normal conditions contribute to the general well-being of man by synthesizing a number of growth factors (vitamins) essential for good nutrition.

The tubercle bacillus (*Mycobacterium tuberculosis*) occurs in many species of animals as well as in man. It has caused a high rate of death and disease for centuries. Although the disease is less frequent and of shorter duration today, it still remains a major cause of death and illness. An outstanding characteristic of these organisms is that they will take an acid-fast stain (this is a special laboratory test). They are extremely slender, nonmotile (nonmoving) rods of variable length. These bacilli differ from most bacteria in having an abundance of fatty material in them. Tubercle bacilli because of their chemical makeup have a hydrophobic (water-repelling) surface. Therefore, they are not wetted readily by watery solutions and are difficult to kill with some chemical agents. (Further discussion will be found on p. 58.)

Spore Formation. Certain types of bacilli (not cocci) are capable through their more complex reproductive cycle of changing into highly resistant bodies called spores. This remarkable property of spore formation is confined to only a *few species* of bacilli, but it is of extreme importance when an attempt is made to render an object sterile, that is, entirely free of living organisms. All spore-forming bacilli are native to the soil, where they exist in the spore state. Many of these are native to the intestinal tract of animals and human beings. Some kinds generally are present in dust and therefore become widely distributed in any environment.

It is fortunate that only a few of these spore-bearing organisms can cause disease. Most of them are harmless saprophytes. The most important pathogenic spore-formers are:

Clostridium tetani, causing tetanus
Clostridium perfringes, causing gas gangrene
Bacillus anthracis, causing anthrax

Some spore-bearing bacilli change to spore forms (sporulate) more rapidly than others. Sporulation is preceded by a period of active multiplication. The effect of the change of the bacilli to spores is a means of preservation of life. Sporulation is a *regular habit of spore-forming bacilli and a part of their normal cycle of development.*

THE PROCESS OF SPORE FORMATION is as follows:

1. Newly germinated rods divide at once into two actively growing bacilli (reproductive phase, Fig. 10).

2. Each bacillus is in an actively growing state (vegetative form, Fig. 11A).

3. With special laboratory staining, one can see a collection of cell content as a spot appears at the end or the center of the rod (condensate form, Fig. 11B).

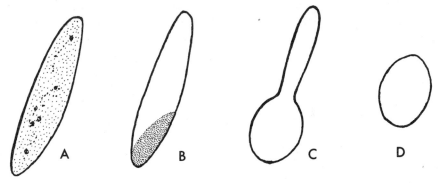

Fig. 11. Process of spore formation: (A) vegetative form; (B) condensate form; (C) endospore form; (D) free spore. For reproductive phase see Figure 10.

4. The spot enlarges until often it has a greater diameter than that of the cell in which it is forming (endospore form, Fig. 11C).

5. The original cell decreases in size, giving up its vital matter to the spore. The spore ruptures from the original cell (which disintegrates) and becomes a free spore (free spore stage, Fig. 11D).

The free bacterial spore, now resembling a seed, is highly resistant to physical or chemical changes that would injure or destroy the original organism. It is capable of germination; that is, it can return to the original growing form with all of the original properties intact when it is placed in a favorable environment.

The vegetative forms of spore formers are *no more resistant* to destruction than nonspore-forming bacilli. However, free spores resist destruction by heat, cold, drying and chemicals to a remarkable degree. Free spores are viable (living) but dormant (sleeping) in a dehydrated state, surrounded by a hard protective shell. Spore germination is the reversal of the process of spore formation.

FUNGI

YEASTS AND MOLDS

Yeasts and molds are two types of fungi; they are microscopic plants without the green coloring matter—chlorophyll—that is peculiar to ordinary plants. The distinction between yeasts and molds is perplexing even to the specialists, the mycologists. We shall consider molds as woolly fungi with long filaments (strands which resemble branches and roots) and yeasts as nonfilamentous fungi. Each of these living forms is much larger than bacterial cells.

Yeasts and molds are distributed widely in nature, and most of them are saprophytes. Yeasts can be found on grapes, other fruit and plants, in soil, milk, river water, dust and throat cultures. Bakers' and brewers' yeast are familiar products. Yeasts give off enzymes which cause chemical changes in sugars called *fermentation,* a process which produces alcohol and carbon dioxide. The action of nonpathogenic yeasts causes dough to rise, beer to foam, holes to form in bread and champagne to bubble.

Molds live in soil and actively decompose organic matter. Familiar to all are the various colored molds on stale bread, jelly, old books, rags, or old leather shoes which have been stored in damp places for some time. Because of the growth of molds, Roquefort, Camembert, and "blue" cheeses have specific aroma, texture and flavor. Penicillin, an outstanding drug discovery, is derived from a mold found in dust and in soil.

Pathogenic yeasts and molds are those which cause "ringworm" and "athlete's foot," thrush and vaginitis, serious poisoning, a fatal form of meningitis, serious skin ulcerations, and often fatal infections of tissues in all parts of the body.

Like bacteria, many yeasts and molds are more helpful than dangerous to human beings.

VIRUSES

A satisfactory definition of a virus cannot yet be made; scientists are still trying to determine their true nature. However, some information about viruses exists although the key to their character has not yet been found:

Viruses are the simplest known forms of life.

There are many different kinds of viruses.

Viruses are much smaller than bacteria and cannot be seen with a standard microscope.

Viruses are able to pass through filters which can hold back bacteria.

Viruses will not grow on artificial laboratory media (i.e., food preparation), but they do grow on living cells. Those that act on bacteria are called bacteriophages.

It is felt that most of the viruses are readily destroyed through sterilization practices and most chemical disinfection routines.

At present viruses are classified according to the diseases they cause; for example, there is a polio virus, a cold virus, a smallpox virus and so on. So far as operating room technology is concerned, the hepatitis virus is the one type against which very careful precautions must be taken. Hepatitis viruses are categorized as being perhaps more resistant to destruction than other viruses, although this has not been proved. The enormous void in present understanding of the nature of hepatitis viruses reinforces the need for strict controls over all aseptic practices.

BODY DEFENSES

The body constantly is being assailed by pathogenic microorganisms. However, it has a number of built-in defense mechanisms that serve to protect it against injury and disease.

Protective Defense Mechanisms

Skin is the first line of defense which protects the entire body surface. Skin normally has some microorganisms living on and within it. These are called *transients* (those which are picked up on objects and washed off with good hygiene) and *residents* (those which live in skin glands and hair follicles). Transient and resident bacteria are considered to be *normal flora;* that is, they ordinarily are found on this particular tissue. When skin is intact, and when the glands are secreting normally, pathogenic bacteria cannot enter the body through the skin to produce disease. Skin acts like a wall to keep out most foreign bacteria. (For further discussion of Skin see p. 89.)

The mucous membrane lining the nose, the mouth, the respiratory, the digestive and the other tracts also has a protective function, although it also harbors normal flora. Foreign bacteria entering the nose, the throat or the digestive system become entangled in the mucus which is secreted by the cells within the membrane. Some of these cells have *cilia* (tiny hair structures) which hold bacteria or sweep them from the body.

Highly acid secretions from cells in the vaginal mucous membrane destroy pathogens that may enter the vagina. Menstrual flow likewise carries away bacteria. The hydrochloric acid of the stomach also kills many microbes that are swallowed.

The eyes are protected by the lubricating action of tears, which have the ability to destroy microorganisms.

Phagocytes, a specialized type of white blood cells, have the ability to engulf and to destroy bacteria which may have invaded the skin. (See Infection.)

Specific Organs. The liver and the stomach each play important roles in the defense of the body. The liver, rich in blood supply, serves to destroy bacterial cells; so does the hydrochloric acid in the stomach, mentioned earlier.

Lymphatic System. Lymph and lymph vessels serve an important protective purpose: the lymph nodes act as filters for the removal of infectious organisms. The enlargement of tonsils in tonsillitis is an example. The lymphatic system also produces antibodies.

Immunity is another defense mechanism of the body which for some diseases can be acquired. When a person previously has encountered certain organisms, specific resistance or immunity is built up by mechanisms in the blood which produce protective substances called antibodies. These antibodies act in one of many ways to kill new invading bacteria, to neutralize bacterial toxins, or to make bacteria more vulnerable to attack by white blood cells. Vaccines and toxoids given by injection confer immunity by scientific means. Immunity to some diseases is acquired naturally. To contract even a mild case of, say, polio can result in total immunity thereafter.

In a healthy body all of these body defenses fight off bacteria effectively. However, injury, fatigue, exposure, chilling, dietary deficiencies and other conditions serve to lower these defenses.

REPAIRING INJURIES

Inflammation is the local tissue reaction of the body to injury or irritation. It is the body's protective and defense mechanism to repair an injury by isolating and eliminating the injuring agent. Usually a helpful process, inflammation plays an important part in fractures, sprains, burns, open wounds and infection.

Causes of Inflammation. Any of the following types of injuring agents may cause inflammation:

1. Trauma, such as a blow or mechanical irritation.
2. Chemicals, such as stings of insects, poison ivy, venom of snakes.
3. Cold or heat.
4. Pathogenic bacteria, such as staphylococci and streptococci.
5. Other agents, such as the rays of the sun, electricity and x-ray.

Signs. Inflammation anywhere in the body is characterized by five distinct symptoms: redness, heat, swelling, pain and disturbance of function. These symptoms occur as a reaction of injured blood vessels and tissues.

When an injury occurs, the blood vessels dilate, thus increasing the blood supply to the injured area and producing the first two signs of *redness* and *heat*. With the dilatation of blood vessels, the walls of the vessels leak, and serum escapes into the tissue. This causes the *swelling*. Swelling exerts pressure on nerve endings, causing *pain,* which in turn results in *disturbance of function.*

While blood vessel changes produce these many signs, white blood cells move through the dilated vessels, through the tissue fluids, and wall off the injured area. Working as scavengers (phagocytes), the white cells ingest dead tissue, particles of foreign matter and bacteria, if present.

As the inflammation subsides, tissues return to normal size, white cells disperse, blood vessels return to normal size, fluids flow away through lymphatics, and if tissues have been destroyed, they are replaced by scar tissue (cicatrix).

In summary, the inflammatory process, which can occur anywhere in the body, results in the dilatation of blood vessels and the mobilization of white cells against the injuring agents.

Infection is bacterial-caused inflammation. As stated above, white cells and body fluids may localize around the injured area, forming a wall and destroying invading organisms. As white cells attack bacteria within the wall, destroyed cells, bacteria and tissue mix with tissue fluid to form *pus. Abscess* formation is a walled-in collection of pus.

Furuncles and carbuncles are common types of abscesses. A *furuncle* (boil) is a collection of pus beneath the skin. A *carbuncle* is a similar but more severe condition in which several abscesses have grown together to form one inflamed area beneath the skin. Abscesses may develop in any part of the body in any type of tissue. However, they are most common in the skin. A common surgical procedure is an I & D (incision and drainage) of an abscess. However, some abscesses grow toward the skin surface and drain spontaneously.

There is danger that body defenses will fail to overcome the invading bacteria. If this occurs, bacteria and their poisons enter the blood stream and spread throughout the body. This serious condition is called *septicemia.*

Bacteria, including pathogens, exist on everything which is not sterilized. When skin or mucous membrane is broken or otherwise irritated, bacteria may invade tissues and produce infection. Whereas one bacterial invasion may result in mild infection, another may be severe. This explains the reason that one infection may be a pimple, another may take the form of a boil, and still another may invade the blood stream.

Healing is a fascinating process wherein most tissues are replaced by scar tissue (a fibrous type of connective tissue). Only a few damaged tissues in the body are capable of replacing themselves in kind. Some of these are bone, kidney tubules

A. FIRST INTENTION (Primary union)

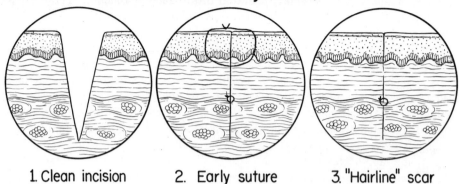

1. Clean incision   2. Early suture   3. "Hairline" scar

B. SECOND INTENTION (Granulation)

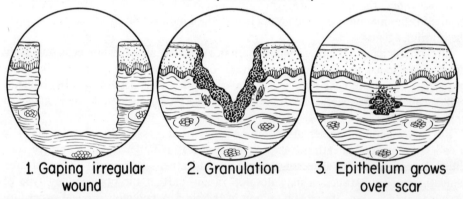

1. Gaping irregular wound   2. Granulation   3. Epithelium grows over scar

Fig. 12. Chronologic course of wound healing by first and second intention. In the final stage of second intention healing it is to be noted that the under side of the epithelium is smooth and serrated as it is normally. (Harkins, H. N., *et al.*: Surgery, Principles and Practice, ed. 2, Fig. 2-1, p. 8, Philadelphia, Lippincott, 1961)

and liver. Other tissues, like brain, heart muscle or eye, are replaced with connective tissue. Wound healing can occur in one of two ways:

1. *First intention.* This also is called *primary union,* in which a clean wound is closed by sutures (stitches), and the tissue walls are approximated (brought together). When healing is complete, a thin scar holds the walls together.

2. *Second intention.* This also is called *secondary union,* in which the wound is not approximated but is left open to heal by granulation tissue from the bottom up. Granulation tissue is a network of fiber cells and capillaries (smallest of blood vessels) which form at the base and along the walls of the wound. As granulation

tissue fills the wound, foreign matter is crowded out, and the wound is covered by skin. A wide irregular scar is usual for these wounds.

REVIEW QUESTIONS:
1. Differentiate between the terms "microbiology" and "biology."
2. What are bacteria?
3. Discuss the meaning of "normal flora."
4. Discuss pathogenicity of bacteria and its significance to your study.
5. What is meant by the term "aseptic"?
6. What kinds of microorganisms most concern us in relation to operating room work? Why?
7. What are the body's normal defenses against bacterial invasion?
8. What factors are necessary to bacterial growth?
9. How does a wound heal?
10. Where in the body can infection occur?

Bibliography

Bryan, A. H., and Bryan, C. G.: Bacteriology, Principles and Practice, ed. 5, College Outline Series, New York, Barnes & Noble, 1954.
Burdon, K. L., and Williams, R. P.: Microbiology, ed. 5, New York, Macmillan, 1964
Frobisher, M., and Sommermeyer, L.: Microbiology for Nurses ed. 11, Philadelphia, Saunders, 1964.
Wheeler, M. F., and Volk, W. A.: Basic Microbiology, Philadelphia, Lippincott, 1964.

CHAPTER 4

PRINCIPLES OF ASEPSIS

DEFINITIONS : THE STERILIZATION PROCESS : CHEMICAL
DISINFECTION : CHEMICAL ANTISEPSIS

DEFINITIONS

Asepsis is a broad term used to describe a series of procedures intended to reduce the possibility of infection in patients and personnel (a = without; sepsis = infection). Many procedures done before, during and after surgery are referred to as "aseptic technics." Asepsis, then, covers a wide area of controlled practices which, if carried out conscientiously, will reduce the incidence of sepsis in patients and personnel. For instance, the *sterilization* of goods and supplies is one aspect of aseptic technic; *disinfection* of the hospital environment is another; *antisepsis* of hands and arms of operating room personnel and the wearing of "scrub" clothes and proper masks are still other facets of this inclusive term.

Sterilization is a process by which *all forms* of living matter are destroyed. (This includes bacteria, viruses, yeasts and molds.) This term is distinguished from *disinfection,* in which liquid chemicals are used to destroy pathogenic bacteria on *inanimate* surfaces, such as floors, furniture and walls. It is distinguished from *antisepsis,* in which liquid chemicals are used to destroy pathogenic bacteria on *animate* surfaces, such as the skin. Finally, it is distinguished from *sanitization,* in which a good cleaning process or boiling water is used to destroy bacteria. Some spores of resistant spore-formers can survive prolonged periods in boiling water. *Sterilization,* then, is a positive term which is applied without qualifying adjectives. It is incorrect to state that a package is "nearly" or "partially" sterile. It is or it is not sterile.

THE STERILIZATION PROCESS

Sterilization is achieved through the use of special equipment and a series of controlled practices utilizing moist heat or dry heat or ethylene oxide gas.

44

MOIST HEAT AS A STERILIZING AGENT

Dressing Sterilizer (standard, gravity displacement apparatus). This is the most popular type of sterilizer used in hospitals today. Moist heat in the form of saturated steam under pressure is the most efficient medium known for the destruction of all forms of microbial life. The equipment necessary is a pressure vessel (like a pressure cooker in its function) called a dressing sterilizer. It is of metal construction and contains two shells to form a jacket and a chamber. More common usage refers to this equipment as an autoclave, although technically an autoclave is a single-shell unit. (Fig. 13)

Steam is generated in a boiler room and piped to each dressing sterilizer; or steam may be obtained from an electric generator mounted beneath the unit or by means of a gas burner located under the unit. Steam is water vapor. When steam contains the maximum amount of water vapor, it is said to be saturated.

When saturated steam enters a sterilizing chamber, it condenses as it contacts cold objects. The condensation causes the liberation of a large amount of heat, simultaneously heating and wetting all of the materials. This is called heating by convection. In this manner the necessary moisture and the heat vital to sterilization are provided. As steam enters the chamber behind the baffle, it is deflected upward. This mechanism aids the normal tendency of steam to rise, since it is twice as light as air. As more steam is admitted to fill the chamber, the air within the chamber and in the wrapped goods is displaced with steam by gravity. The air which is forced out passes through the sedimentation screen to the waste line, which is guarded by a thermostatic trap. During the displacement of air and the flow of condensate (steam that turns to water) through the line, the bellows within the trap remains open. When pure saturated steam has filled the chamber and flows out the line, the bellows seats itself and opens only periodically throughout the cycle.

The process by which bacteria are destroyed when they are subjected to moist heat is not clearly understood. However, an accepted theory is that moist heat causes the coagulation of essential protein or enzyme-protein systems within bacterial cells.

There are some *fundamental principles* underlying the use of steam as a sterilizing agent: (1) Steam under pressure is used rather than steam at atmospheric pressure so that a higher temperature may be attained. (2) Pressure *by itself* has no effect on the killing power of steam. Nonpressure steam has a maximum temperature of 212° F. and is of *no* value in the sterilization of surgical supplies. (3) Bacterial spores are recognized as the most resistant of living organisms in their ability to withstand external destructive forces. Carefully documented studies on the microbicidal effect of high temperature moist heat provide significant information. With control of wrapping materials, size and packaging of bundles, and placement in sterilizers, an effective standard cycle is 250–254° F. (equivalent to 15–17 pounds pressure per square inch) for an exposure period of 30 minutes. (4) To be effective, saturated steam under pressure must be able to surround, to contact, to envelop or to penetrate every portion of every object to be sterilized. Therefore it is necessary that linens be packaged appropriately, and that wrapped or unwrapped instruments be cleaned and opened (disengaged) before sterilization.

Despite its acknowledged efficiency, this type of sterilizer has *some limitations:* (1) There is no valid way of determining that the air elimination from the chamber during the cycle is complete. Overloading a sterilizer, improper placement or too tightly wrapped goods may trap air which will decrease or nullify the effectiveness of the process. (2) The unit takes 15 to 25 minutes to build up to sterilization temperature, 30 minutes for the exposure, and 20 to 30 minutes to dry a load. The complete process is time-consuming. (3) Steam is not effective in the sterilization of anhydrous (without water) substances such as oils, powders or greases. (4) Steam is not suitable for the sterilization of heat-sensitive items such as some plastic materials and carbon steel instruments.

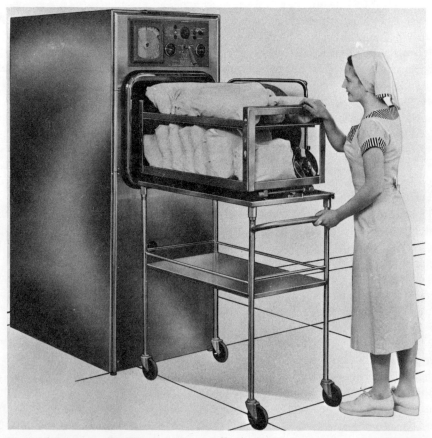

Fig. 13. Standard dressing sterilizer, gravity displacement type. (AMSCO, American Sterilizer Company, Erie, Pa.)

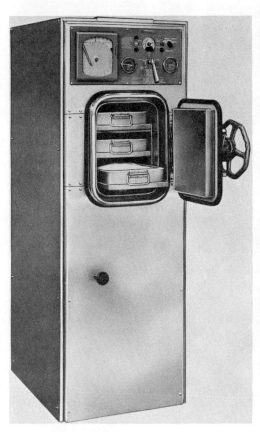

Fig. 14. High speed instrument sterilizer. (AMSCO, American Sterilizer Company)

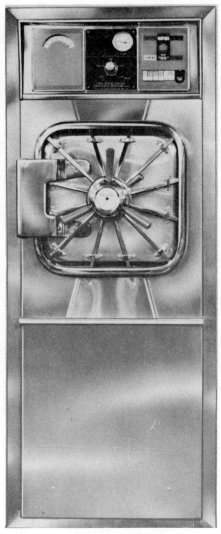

Fig. 15. Instrument washer-sterilizer. (Wilmot Castle Company, Rochester, N.Y.)

Instrument Sterilizer. Common usage refers to these units as high-speed or flash sterilizers. The design and the operation are identical with those of the dressing sterilizers except that instrument sterilizers generally have a smaller chamber capacity (to permit them to function rapidly), and they have been constructed to permit temperatures of 270–272° F. Scientific evidence proves that as the temperature is increased, the exposure period can be decreased. (Fig. 14)

This apparatus was developed for emergency sterilization of unwrapped instru-

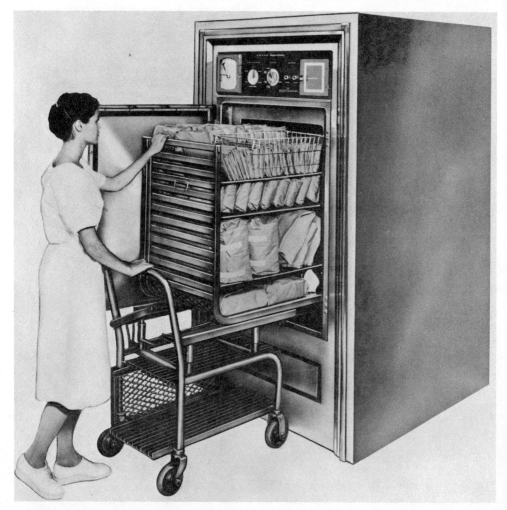

Fig. 16. A load is going into the high vacuum Vacamatic sterilizer. (AMSCO, American Sterilizer Company)

ments when the need was felt for a fast method of sterilizing individual instruments or sets. The standardized safe cycle is for 3 minutes at 270° F. The entire process from build-up of temperature to delivery of sterile items takes about 5 minutes.

Instrument Washer-Sterilizer. This unit is designed as a safe technic for the terminal cleaning and the sterilizing of instruments immediately after surgery. Dirty instruments are opened so that all surfaces are exposed, and then they are put in perforated trays. The trays are placed in the sterilizer, appropriate detergent is added, and superheated water removes soil and debris. This machine is equipped with automatic controls. The cycle takes about 20 minutes and reaches a temperature of 270° F. (Fig. 15)

If the washing cycle is eliminated by a simple turn of a switch, this unit can be used as an instrument sterilizer.

High Vacuum Sterilizer. One of the stated major disadvantages of the dressing sterilizer is the inability to predict accurately the time necessary for complete air removal from the materials and from the chamber. High vacuum sterilizers are relatively new units which eliminate this problem as well as others associated with the traditional gravity displacement units.

The cycle is designed to provide a prevacuum and a postvacuum phase. The total time is about 15 minutes. By eliminating the temperature build-up lag of the other units, the sterilization temperature is 275° F. Equipped with automatic controls and monitored by charts which indicate and record pressures and temperatures, this unit is designed for 3 different cycles in a single unit. High vacuum sterilizers are rapidly replacing gravity displacement sterilizers because the system is safe, reliable and rapid.

DRY HEAT STERILIZER (HOT AIR)

The use of a dry heat oven is limited to the sterilization of those articles which cannot withstand the corrosive action of steam, such as carbon steel instruments and anhydrous substances like oil, grease and powder. With the introduction of effective gas sterilizers and with better packaging of many commercial items, dry heat sterilizers are being used with less frequency in hospitals.

The design of the unit is like that of an insulated household oven, but the sterilizer usually contains a fan to circulate the air evenly and to hasten heating. The whole process is time-consuming, for it takes almost an hour to build up to 320° F., the sterilization temperature. Depending on the type of load, the materials are exposed for 1 or 2 hours, and a 30–60-minute cooling period follows. Death of bacteria is much slower in this method than in the method using moist heat, and higher temperatures are necessary for long periods. The heat in the unit is attained by conduction, like the heat that emanates from a radiator. The dry heat process literally bakes the protoplasm of the bacterial cells. (Figs. 17, 18)

ETHYLENE OXIDE GAS STERILIZER

This is the latest method of sterilization. Available from a number of manufacturers in various sizes, this equipment uses a mixture of ethylene oxide gas and other gases as the sterilant. The concentration of ethylene oxide varies with different equipment, but all the manufacturers have succeeded in rendering a highly flammable gas both safe and effective. It is assumed that this gas kills bacteria by reacting on the chemicals in the protein of the cell, making these cells unable to fulfill their

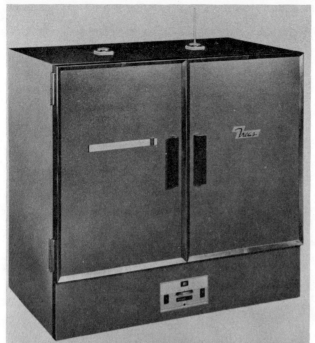

Fig. 17. Freas dry heat sterilizer. (Precision Scientific Co., Chicago)

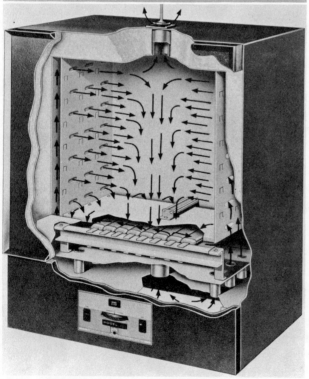

Fig. 18. Cross section of the dry heat sterilizer. (Precision Scientific Co., Chicago)

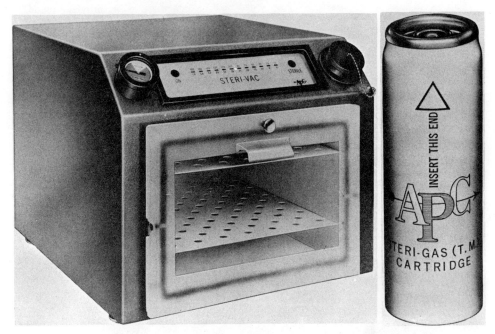

Fig. 19. (*Left*) Ethylene oxide Steri-Vac sterilizer. (*Right*) Cartridge of ethylene oxide which is inserted in the upper right opening of the Steri-Vac sterilizer. (Advanced Products Corp., Framingham, Mass.)

biological function. Equipped with automatic controls, the various units take from 48 minutes to 4 hours to complete a cycle from room temperature to 140° F.

Although this equipment is not intended to replace sterilization by saturated steam, it is particularly useful for the sterilization of nonheat-stable items such as carbon steel eye instruments, certain plastic materials, lens-carrying instruments, electrocautery cords and tips, burrs, rubber parts of anesthesia machines and rubber gloves. When absorbent materials such as rubber goods are sterilized by gas, they must be aerated. Placing such goods on a shelf after sterilization for 24 hours will permit the absorbed gas to be eliminated. (Figs. 19, 20)

MEANS OF VERIFYING THE STERILIZATION PROCESS

Rigid sterilization controls are imposed on all commercially prepared sterile items. The law requires that whatever the method of sterilization, each load must be tested bacteriologically. The entire contents of each load is impounded (quarantined) for the period of incubation and not released for distribution until the efficiency of the cycle has been assured. This time interval is 7 to 14 days.

Unfortunately, hospitals cannot follow this plan. For hospital-sterilized materials it is not possible to assemble either the storage facilities for large volumes of goods

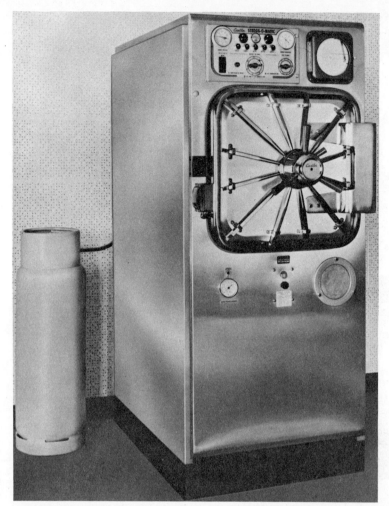

Fig. 20. Castle ethylene oxide sterilizer. (*Continued on facing page*)

or the massive inventory of raw materials required. For these reasons every effort must be made to avoid sterilization failures.

Education is the first important prerequisite. No one should be entrusted with the responsibilities of preparing and processing materials, loading or operating sterilizers until there is repeated evidence of a thorough knowledge of the specific details of the whole process. Although manufacturers of modern equipment have provided a number of automatic features, the possibilities of human error are ever-present. Sound education and supervised practice are important for all personnel handling sterilizers.

Graphic Charts. Recording thermometers should be standard equipment on all steam sterilizers. When properly installed and used, they graphically record the temperature in the discharge line and the duration of each exposure. The chart

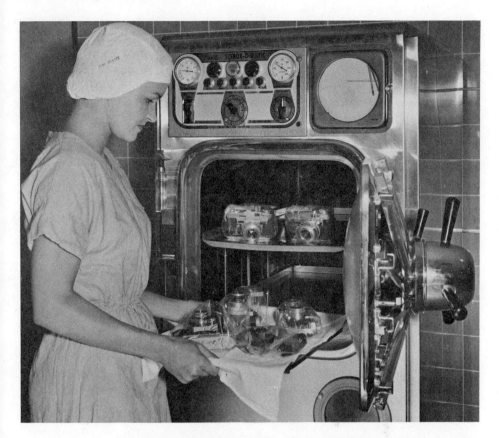

Fig. 20. (*Cont.*) Close-up showing loading of the Castle ethylene oxide sterilizer. (Wilmot Castle Company, Rochester, N.Y.)

thus created serves as a safety sentinel to assure maintenance of temperature during the entire cycle. The charts should be dated, changed daily, and kept for reference for about 6 months.

Culture Tests. The most reliable method to determine the efficiency of sterilizers is the controlled use of known quantities of heat-resistant spore-forming organisms. Most hospital laboratories are not equipped to prepare these tests reliably. A few commercial suppliers sell valid testing materials in hermetically sealed ampules as well as on filter paper strips. The resistant test organism for checking steam sterilization methods is *Bacillus stearothermophilus;* for gas sterilization *Bacillus subtilis* or its variant *Bacillus globigii* is used. Minimum standards of the Joint Commission on Hospital Accreditation require bacteriologic testing of each sterilizer at least once a month. Many hospitals check their equipment every week.

Swab culturing of sterile goods to attest sterility is limited in its usefulness. In this method bacteriologic controls are absent, and one cannot determine what organisms were present before sterilization.

Other Aids and Their Value. *Heat-sensitive Tape.* Packages wrapped for sterilization may be secured with a small piece of color-change tape that is fashioned with a tab for easy removal. When subjected to sterilization conditions (there is a special tape for steam sterilization and another one for gas sterilization), markings appear on the tape to indicate that the goods have been through a sterilization process. The markings do *not* indicate sterility.

Within recent years a variety of specially treated paper envelopes have similar ink markings that respond to high temperature moist heat. It should be re-emphasized that the color change or the imprints that appear following the process of sterilization do not attest sterility.

Indicators. A highly controversial issue is the use of chemical sterilization indicators, sometimes called "telltales." Most authorities agree that their actual worth

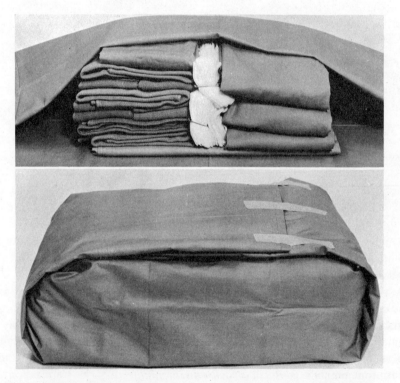

Fig. 21. (*Top*) In preparing a pack for sterilization use only freshly laundered fabrics. See text for proper folding and placement of linens and dressings. (*Bottom*) Finished pack should be no larger than 12″ x 12″ x 20″ and should weigh no more than 12 pounds. (AMSCO, American Sterilizer Company, Erie, Pa.)

is questionable. These indicators do show generally that a load has passed through a sterilizer. If indicators are used, they should be placed in the center of the largest and most densely wrapped bundle in the load.

EQUIPMENT PACKAGING AND LOADING THE STERILIZER

In most hospitals the preparation, the loading and the sterilization of materials are functions of the Central Service Department. However, since operating room personnel and others use the sterilized products, it is important to have sound knowledge and experience regarding the whole process. The key to safe performance of steam sterilization lies in the ability of moisture and heat to envelop and to penetrate every portion of every object to be sterilized. Specific products are described in Chapter 5, and broad principles are discussed here.

Packaging. The most popular type of wrapper and draping material is 140-thread muslin used in double thickness. This fabric has been shown to be effective in providing protection against contact contamination in handling sterile packages, it serves as a good dust filter, and it guards against entry of vermin or insects. In addition, it is readily permeated by moist heat and gas during sterilization processes.

Freshly laundered muslin should be used, since it contains the normal moisture content peculiar to the particular fibers. This moisture is essential to avoid superheating of fabrics during steam sterilization. Superheating of textiles causes a loss of tensile strength, charring and deterioration of the fabric. It is a condition that results from an increase of the temperature of steam over that of saturated steam. It occurs when dehydrated fabrics are subjected repeatedly to steam sterilization.

On an illuminated table in the laundry (or in a specially designed Pack Room) clean linen should be inspected carefully for holes, tears or other damage that would interfere with the protective function of the material.

Heavy woven fabrics, canvas and some types of duck or twill should not be used, because tightly woven fibers will retard the transmission of steam and thereby nullify the sterilization process.

The substitution of muslin wrappers by paper products is increasing. This apparent trend is acceptable, provided that the selected paper is capable of passing steam freely; is devoid of holes, cracks or tears; will not rupture readily; is easy to handle; and is economically feasible to use.

Wrappers should be large enough to envelop the articles easily, and open wrappers should be large enough to serve also as a sterile surface. The packaging should be done securely, but it should not be squeezed tightly since this may retard steam penetration. Single or multiple pieces of material, gowns, half-sheets and laparotomy sheets are fanfolded or loosely rolled to provide the least possible resistance for the passage of steam. Metalware is not included within linen packs, because their presence would cause deflection of steam and ineffective penetration. (Fig. 21)

In packaging goods for ethylene oxide sterilization, it is necessary that each

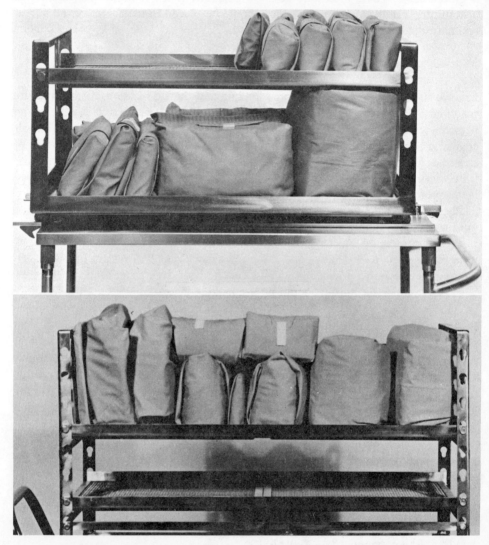

Fig. 22. (*Top*) In loading an autoclave place all packs on edge. Arrange load in sterilizer so that steam can get all around every pack. Do not overload the chamber. (*Bottom*) In putting two layers of packs on one shelf, place the upper layer crosswise on the bottom layer. (AMSCO, American Sterilizer Co.)

article be given prior cleaning. A variety of wrapping materials are suitable, ranging from special papers and muslin cloth to some types of flexible plastic films. However, some plastics are *not* suitable packaging materials. The wrapping materials selected must be permeable to gas and moisture, relatively inexpensive, flexible and easy to wrap and seal, sufficiently strong to withstand handling, and capable of being stored without deterioration under various conditions of temperature and humidity.

Loading. In loading articles in a sterilizer, the goal is to remove air quickly and to permit free passage of steam throughout the load. For these reasons, packs and other wrapped articles are placed on edge rather than flat side up to permit steam to pass from the top of the chamber through multiple folds in the pack toward the bottom.

Packs are arranged in loose contact with each other, and the upper layer is placed crosswise over the lower layer. In this manner free circulation of steam (and elimination of air) passes through all portions of the load. (Fig. 22)

Solid, nonporous articles, i.e., jars, test tubes and basins, should be so arranged in the load that if they were filled with water, the water would drain out. This loading principle provides a horizontal escape for air and permits steam to enter solid objects.

This discussion should make it obvious that it is possible for sterilization equipment to function very efficiently, but that *unsterile* products may be the result. This possibility points up the reason for understanding and following the principles of wrapping and loading as they affect the sterilization process.

CHEMICAL DISINFECTION

DEFINITION

Chemical disinfection means to destroy by the use of chemicals, or at least to render harmless, microorganisms that are capable of producing disease or infection. When an article needed for use in surgery cannot be sterilized by autoclaving, other methods must be used to make the article bacteriologically safe. One such method is chemical disinfection. For example, the high temperature of the autoclave would reduce the adhesive properties of the lens cement in endoscopes. It is therefore necessary to use other methods of disinfecting such instruments, and chemical disinfection is one of the ways to accomplish this objective.

PURPOSE

The basic purpose of chemical disinfection is to make the instrument, the article or the equipment bacteriologically safe for use in surgery.

Gas sterilization, using ethylene oxide (mixed with other gases), is effective in some instances for those articles of supply that cannot be autoclaved, or that should not be subjected to chemicals for disinfection purposes. The development of new model gas sterilizers has increased the availability and the use of this method in hospitals. However, the cost of these units and the time needed for the completion of the sterilizing cycle may present a problem and be prohibitive in some situations.

ACTION

Like steam, the selected liquid chemicals destroy microorganisms by solidifying the protein substance (cytoplasm) of the microbial cell. Some chemicals do this rapidly in 5 to 10 minutes, whereas others take longer.

Major Conditions. Chemical disinfection achieves its effectiveness—that is, the destruction of the organisms intended to be eliminated—only when certain conditions are met. These conditions are as follows:

1. The object must be clean prior to disinfection. Dirt, oil, grease and organic debris such as blood, pus or serum must be removed, since these substances harbor microorganisms and protect them from the action of the disinfecting agent.

2. Complete submersion is essential. Every surface of the article to be disinfected by the solution must be reached by the solution. In the case of hollow tubelike instruments or tubing, air bubbles must be released. This can be done by gently moving the article back and forth 2 or 3 times in the solution. In the case of hollow tubelike instruments, tilt the article to allow air bubbles to escape. In disinfecting a long coil of plastic tubing, it may be necessary to force the chemical solution through the tube with a syringe until all air bubbles have escaped. Hinged instruments should be open so that the solution can contact all surfaces of the instrument.

3. The desired concentration of the solution must be maintained. Smooth-surfaced metal instruments must be washed thoroughly and *dried*. If they are immersed while still wet with water, the concentration of the solution will be diluted, thereby reducing its effectiveness or destroying it.

When "Quat" solutions are used in a basin lined with gauze (such as for cystoscopes), the gauze attracts the basic components of the solution; thereby the concentration is diluted, and this practice becomes unsafe. With continuing research and development, this may change in time, but today this statement is valid.

Criteria of Choice of Chemical. When these major conditions are met, the choice of the chemical or combination of chemicals is determined on the basis of several factors:

1. Specification—the type of organisms to be killed or rendered harmless (such as vegetative organisms, tubercle bacilli, spores or viruses).

2. Stability of the solution—the length of time necessary to do the job.

3. Concentration of the solution.

4. Cost of the solution.

5. Practicability of the solution (full-strength carbolic acid solution kills microorganisms quickly, but a drop of it on the skin of the person using it will burn).

6. The temperature needed for effective disinfection; room or higher temperature.

Here we are concerned primarily with the elimination of four main categories of microorganisms that may cause disease and infections. These are:

1. Vegetative organisms (ordinary bacteria such as the staphylococci).

2. Tubercle bacilli (which cause tuberculosis infections).

3. Spores (which cause gas gangrene and tetanus).

4. Viruses (which are responsible for several types of postoperative infections).

The most difficult of these organisms to kill with chemical disinfectants are spores (see Chap. 3). Next are the tubercle bacilli. Vegetative organisms are the most susceptible to chemical disinfection and the easiest to deal with effectively.

Recent research has demonstrated that viruses fall into two rather sharply distinct groups with respect to resistance to germicides. This is on the basis of whether or not they contain lipid (a substance resembling fats in appearance and solubility but containing elements other than those which make up true fats). Therefore, some are resistant to certain chemical disinfectants, namely, the "Quats," phenolics and isopropyl alcohol.

USES OF CHEMICAL DISINFECTION

Some specific items used in surgery cannot be steam sterilized. Although some of them might be capable of withstanding ethylene oxide sterilization, there are still many hospitals that do not have access to this method of sterilization. Therefore, chemical disinfection must be instituted to insure the safety of the patient during surgery.

Lensed Instruments (endoscopic instruments). When available, ethylene oxide gas sterilization is recommended. In its absence immersion in a "Quat" solution such as Urolicide or Aqueous Zephiran may be used, but such solutions lack tuberculocidal or sporicidal action. A new product, Cidex (activated glutaraldehyde), is an effective agent for lensed instruments; it does have both tuberculocidal and sporicidal action, and it does not injure the lenses or their adhesive properties. This solution is aqueous and includes an antirust agent.

The lensed instrument first must be cleaned thoroughly, the lumen (inside surfaces) flushed, all detachable parts separated from the scope, and lights checked to be certain they are functioning. Complete immersion of every part of the instrument is mandatory. All the accessories used also must be submitted to the same immersion time.

Alcohol-formalin or alcohol solutions should be avoided as agents for the disinfection of lensed instruments. Solutions containing these chemicals damage the adhesive materials which cement the lens into place and cause loosening and fogging of the lens, necessitating repair of the instrument before it can be used again by the physician.

Polyethylene Tubing. All tubing must be thoroughly cleaned, the lumen flushed, and all air bubbles released. The solution used for disinfection must contact all surfaces of the article that is being immersed. Immersion for 10 minutes in 70 per cent ethyl alcohol is adequate for tuberculocidal effect. However, if storage is desired, long exposure in alcohol will in time cause hardening and swelling of the tubing. A "Quat" solution can be used for the storage of polyethylene *after* the immersion in alcohol. (It must be remembered that the mere immersion of such tubing in the "Quat" solution alone, no matter how long or how concentrated the solution, will not produce a tuberculocidal effect.) A 20-minute immersion time does eliminate vegetative organisms if the article is free from air bubbles and clean before it is put into the solution.

Transfer Forceps. The term "transfer forceps" applies to the instrument used to remove sterile items of supply from one sterile source to a sterile surface. The items transferred may be from sterile containers and packages, from a steam sterilizer or from chemical disinfectant solutions. It must be remembered that the basic strength of the solution in the forceps container may be diluted by other solutions from which the forceps have transferred sterile items, and the dilution consequently will result in decreased bacteriological effectiveness.

In the care of transfer forceps it has been found that weekly autoclaving of the forceps and its container (after thorough soap and water cleansing) and refilling the container with a fresh solution of the desired chemical disinfectant constitute a safe method.

Any solution used for the purpose of disinfecting these forceps should have sporicidal action. Since the forceps are stainless steel, as are the containers in which they repose, an alcohol-formalin or Cidex solution meets this requirement.

Some institutions which have light surgery schedules rather than the 24-hour-a-day schedules maintained in many large medical centers routinely reprocess (autoclave and refill with fresh solution) transfer forceps and containers daily at the end of the operating room schedule. In any situation there should be sterile forceps available for any emergency that might arise. Routines for this usually are set up by the operating room supervisor. For that matter, it is important that a routine-care procedure be instituted in every operating room for the processing of *all* equipment and supplies.

Summary. We have specifically spoken of the chemical disinfection of some items of supply for surgery that cannot be steam sterilized. The many changes in the composition of supplies and articles used in surgery require that all operating room personnel be constantly alert and continue to learn. Each of these new items include instructions, recommendations and information about their use, purchase, care and action. Reliable manufacturers provide documented evidence of the effectiveness of each of their products.

SPECIFIC CHEMICAL DISINFECTANTS

There are many chemical solutions available today for the purpose of disinfection. Only a few of them will be named here, and the use of chemical disinfectants should not be limited to these. However, careful evaluation of each product should be made before any is accepted as the agent for use in an operating room for a specific purpose. Because an individual hospital cannot possibly do research on every product to determine the validity of the manufacturer's claims, chemical disinfectants must be judged on known merits and by the reputation of the company producing them.

No one chemical disinfectant can be used in all types of situations. The composition of the item to be disinfected, the kind and the type of organism which needs to be eliminated, and the properties of the chemical solution must be considered when a selection is made. A solution that could kill the microorganisms present also could be completely destructive to the item being disinfected.

Some of the more commonly used disinfectants are as follows:

Ethyl Alcohol 70–95%

Advantages	Disadvantages	Uses
Kills vegetative organisms, tubercle bacilli and some viruses within 5 minutes of immersion time	Has no sporicidal action	Polyethylene tubing for immediate use: 10-minute immersion
Easily available	Rusts metal unless 0.2% sodium nitrite is added to prevent the formation of rust	Sharp-edged instruments (such as for eye surgery) which cannot be autoclaved
Reasonable in cost	Causes hardening and swelling of polyethylene if used as a storage solution	Electrical cords. A thorough alcohol wipe is a more effective means of chemical disinfection for cords (such as bronchoscope cords) which cannot be autoclaved than a 30-minute immersion in a less effective chemical solution, such as an aqueous "Quat" solution.
	Cannot be used for lensed instruments because it loosens the adhesive used to fixate the lenses and will cause fogging of the lenses in endoscopic instruments	

Alcohol 70%-Formalin 20%

Advantages	Disadvantages	Uses
Sporicidal in 3 hours	A solution containing formalin is prone to be absorbed to a certain degree by porous substances, such as rubber tubing.	Pre-autoclaved transfer forceps and needles can be immersed safely and stored in the solution in closed containers.
Tuberculocidal and effective against vegetative organisms in 5 minutes	Must have a rust-preventative added: 0.2% sodium nitrite will prevent rust forming on metal that is immersed.	
Inexpensive		
Readily available through hospital pharmacies	Cannot be used on skin or mucous membrane because of its toxicity. For this reason it must be thoroughly rinsed off the surface of each item immersed before the item can be used in surgery (such as suture tubes, instruments, or other items transferred by forceps to the sterile field).	
	Cannot be used for lensed instruments, polyethylene tubing, rubber or porous substances	

Aqueous "Quat" Solutions
(Quaternary Ammonium Compounds)

Advantages	Disadvantages	Uses
Effective against vegetative organisms within 20 minutes of immersion Inexpensive	Not effective against free spores or tubercle bacilli Must be used with an understanding of its limitations. The use of a basin lined with gauze is unsafe because the gauze fibers attract the chemical of the solution, and thereby the concentration is diluted.	Lensed instruments Shellac and web catheters which cannot be autoclaved Agent in which to store polyethylene tubing after it has been immersed in alcohol for 10 minutes

Phenolics

Advantages	Disadvantages	Uses
Safe for conductive tile floors and for conductive wheels Effective against vegetative organisms and tubercle bacilli when properly applied with mechanical scrubbing	Enteroviruses (ECHO, polio, Coxsackie) are resistant to the phenolics.	Germicide cleanser for floors, furniture, large equipment, and for washing down walls and floors

Some of the acceptable brand name products are:
1. Tergisyl
2. Ves-phene

These two products are detergent-germicides in which the active agent is less concentrated than it is in the counterpart germicide (e.g., Ves-phene versus Staphene). In the concentrations of these products (2%) tuberculocidal action is poor. Consequently, concentrations of 2 times or 3 times the regular strength should be used when tuberculocidal effect is desired.[1]

3. 1% Amphyl*
4. 1% O-syl*

The advantages, the disadvantages and the uses in operating room nursing practice are the same as those listed above for phenolics in general.

[1] Earle H. Spaulding, Ph.D., Professor and Head of the Department of Microbiology, School of Medicine, Temple University Medical Center.
* If used for metal, 0.5 per cent sodium bicarbonate must be added to prevent rusting.

Iodine Preparations

Advantages	Disadvantages	Uses
Kills vegetative organisms in 10 minutes Tuberculocidal in 20 minutes High fungicidal efficiency	Must be carefully measured to ensure correct concentration Solution is unstable and requires frequent changing to remain fresh and effective.	Cleaning of floors, walls, furniture

ADVANTAGES	DISADVANTAGES	USES
Cleans and disinfects in one operation	In the use of any solution containing iodine, the percentage of available iodine is the key to its bacteriologic effectiveness. Therefore, the concentration is critical. If the solution changes color due to dilution, it must be discarded.	
Nonstaining		
Noninsulating film residue		
Nonirritating to hands of personnel		
	When used as a chemical disinfectant, the available iodine could exert itself on inert or organic material and lose its germicidal effect.	

CIDEX
(Activated Glutaraldehyde)

ADVANTAGES	DISADVANTAGES	USES
Sporicidal in 3 hours	Porosity of polyethylene tubing causes a certain amount of absorption of the chemical and may cause irritation of tissues; it should not be used for porous materials.	Lensed instruments (such as cystoscopes, endoscopic instruments of all kinds)
Tuberculocidal in 10 minutes		Transfer forceps and containers after they have been autoclaved
Effective against vegetative organisms in 5 minutes		Smooth-surfaced metal instruments which cannot be autoclaved
	Items immersed in this solution must be rinsed thoroughly before use in surgery.	Web and shellac catheters
	May be corrosive to metal if used as a prolonged storage solution	Cords for bronchoscopes, etc., when they cannot be autoclaved
	Once activated, the solution is effective for a maximum of 2 weeks.	Most anesthesia equipment: face masks, etc.

GERMICIDAL FOGGING

During the past year, there has been an increase in the number of hospitals investigating various forms of spraying or fogging machines as a means to distribute a disinfectant vapor. There is evidence that the use of such machines has grown considerably during this period and many hospitals are now relying on fogging periodically as an additional tool for terminal disinfection.[2]

The use of fogging with the new technics that are being developed eventually may become common operating room practice and change the usual routine approach to

[2] Chemical specialties, reprinted from Soap and Chemical Specialties, March 1964.

room disinfection used today to something quite different and perhaps more effective. However, the use of fogging technics is still in the preliminary stages.

CHEMICAL ANTISEPSIS

DEFINITION

Chemical antisepsis is the process of applying chemical agents or compounds to the *skin* of patients or members of the surgical team to eliminate or prevent the growth of microorganisms.

PURPOSE

The basic purpose is to destroy or to render harmless the pathogenic bacteria found on animate surfaces.

Since skin cannot be sterilized, and many chemical compounds otherwise used for the disinfection of inanimate objects in surgery are toxic or harmful to the skin, the chemicals employed for the purpose of antisepsis must be selected carefully, depending on the action desired.

SPECIFIC ANTISEPTICS

Some of the more commonly used antiseptics are as follows:

ETHYL ALCOHOL 70–95%

ADVANTAGES	DISADVANTAGES	USES
Nontoxic to skin	Irritating to mucous membranes	Swab for skin disinfection prior to hypodermic, intramuscular or intravenous injections
Easily available		
Reasonable in cost		
Effective against many resident bacteria normally found on skin surfaces		Skin preparation before a surgical incision is made, following the application of the usual skin scrub (see pp. 159, 162, 163, Chap. 8)

Iodine Complexes
(Povidone-Iodine, Polyvinylpyrrolidone or PVP-I)

Advantages	Disadvantages	Uses
Reduces postoperative infections by use of spray after surgery is completed, because it reduces the number of skin bacteria	In the use of any solution containing iodine, the percentage of available iodine is the key to its bacteriological effectiveness.	PVP-I hand scrub for members of the surgical team
Little or no skin sensitivity has been demonstrated. Nonirritating to skin	When used as an antiseptic, the available iodine could exert itself on inert and organic material and lose its germicidal effect.	Preoperative preparation of the patient's skin
Has both a high fungicidal and fungistatic efficiency		Spray following skin preparation for surgery reduces organisms on the surface of the skin at the operative site. Usually it is used following a skin scrub with an agent containing G-11 (hexachlorophene).
		Spray following surgery on the incision and adjacent skin reduces postoperative infections.
		May be used as an effective vaginal douche for many strains of bacteria causing vaginal abnormalities

Aqueous "Quat" Solutions
(Quaternary Ammonium Compounds)

Advantages	Disadvantages	Uses
Nontoxic to tissue	Not effective against free spores or tubercle bacilli	Can be used for vaginal preparation before surgery
Good surface tension depressants (i.e., greater wetting ability, permitting better penetration and distribution of the solution)		Can be used as an arm spray after the hand scrub
Does not irritate mucous membranes or skin		

Review Questions:
1. Differentiate the meaning of the following terms: sterilization, antisepsis, disinfection.
2. Why is the boiling water method considered to be sanitization rather than sterilization?
3. How many sterilization methods are in use? Name them.
4. How does the high vacuum sterilizer differ from a standard steam sterilizer?
5. What is the significance of wrapping and loading procedures in relation to standard steam sterilization methods?

6. Describe the differences between a high-speed sterilizer and an instrument-washer sterilizer.
7. When would one use an ethylene oxide sterilizer?
8. How are chemical indicators different from bacteriologic controls?
9. Why are tightly packaged bundles unsuitable for steam sterilization?
10. What would be the sterilization method of choice for a cystoscope?
11. Explain the various ways in which the concentration of a chemical solution may be changed. Does a change in the concentration affect bacteriologic efficiency of a chemical solution? How?
12. Under what conditions do chemical disinfectants achieve their greatest effectiveness?
13. What factors must be considered in the selection of a chemical disinfectant for use in the operating room?
14. Why is alcohol-formalin or alcohol not used as a disinfectant for lensed instruments?
15. Under what conditions is chemical disinfection used in surgery?
16. Differentiate chemical disinfection from chemical antisepsis.

Bibliography

Guide to Standards for Microbial Control Processing of Hospital Supplies and Equipment, Research and Technical Projects Divisions of the American Sterilizer Co., Erie, Pa.

Joress, S. M.: A study of disinfection of the skin, Ann. Surg. 155:296–304, February 1962.

Perkins, J. J.: Principles and Methods of Sterilization, Springfield, Ill., Thomas, 1956.

Reddish, G. F.: Antiseptics, Disinfectants, Germicides, and Physical Sterilization, Philadelphia, Lea & Febiger, 1954.

Shelanski, H. A., and Shelanski, M. V.: PVP-iodine, history, toxicity and therapeutic uses, J. Int. Coll. Surg. 25:727–734, 1956.

Spaulding, E. H.: Chemical Disinfection of Medical and Surgical Materials, Philadelphia, Temple University Medical Center.

————: Recommendations for Chemical Disinfection of Medical and Surgical Materials (lecture presented at Seton Hall College of Medicine and Dentistry), reprinted by Ethicon, Inc., Somerville, N.J.

————: Principles and application of chemical disinfection, A.O.R.N.J. 1:36–46, May–June 1963.

————: Chemical disinfection in the hospital, J. Hosp. Research 3:1–25, January 1965.

Spaulding, E. H., and Emmons, E. K.: Chemical disinfection, Am. J. Nurs. 58:1238–1242, 1958.

Stonehill, A. A., et al.: Buffered glutaraldehyde, Am. J. Hosp. Pharm. 20:458–465, 1963.

Walter, C. W.: The Aseptic Treatment of Wounds, New York, Macmillan, 1948.

CHAPTER 5

THE NATURE, THE CARE AND THE PREPARATION OF SUPPLIES

SURGICAL INSTRUMENTS : SUTURE MATERIAL : NEEDLES :

GLASSWARE : SOLUTIONS : RUBBER GOODS : PLASTIC

MATERIALS : ELECTRICAL EQUIPMENT : RADIUM AND

RADIOISOTOPES : LENGTH OF TIME SUPPLIES REMAIN STERILE

SURGICAL INSTRUMENTS

Surgical instruments are costly surgeons' tools which are used to help to heal patients. As such, they should be treated as precious jewels. Mishandling and abuse of instruments must be avoided. Most surgical instruments are made of quality stainless steel by reliable manufacturers. This is not to say that they will not stain. The finest quality of stainless steel instruments will stain and will be otherwise damaged unless they are handled and processed with meticulous care based on understanding.

All instruments must be sterilized following each operation. This is called *terminal sterilization*. Processing them through a pressure washer-sterilizer makes them safe for personnel to handle and to inspect. Placing the instruments within a good sonic energy cleaner will remove any remaining debris in box locks or serrations. Thereafter, rinsing and drying are important considerations.

If this equipment is lacking, terminal sterilization can be accomplished by placing opened instruments in a bath of trisodium phosphate solution and subjecting them to sterilization for 45 minutes at 250° F. (The longer exposure period is to permit the sterilization through a large volume of water.) Care must be taken to avoid burns of the hands or the arms due to hot liquids. Inspection of instruments and hand-scrubbing with a soft-bristled brush should follow.

Whatever method is used, instruments first must be thoroughly cleaned so that they are free from organic debris, grease or oil, which will interfere with sterilization. After being rinsed and dried, they may be either stored for future use or reassembled in another set ready for sterilization. If the set is wrapped in double-thickness muslin, it should be sterilized at 250° F. for 30 minutes. Such packaged sets, with instruments opened, may be sterilized also in high vacuum sterilizers. Unwrapped assembled sets may be subjected to the standard autoclave for 15 minutes at 250° F. or to the high speed instrument sterilizer for 3 minutes at 270° F.

ULTRASONIC CLEANER OR SONIC ENERGY UNIT

Before any sterilization process is used, all objects must be clean, that is, free from dirt, debris, oil and grease. These contaminants can form a protective coating on organisms and prevent their destruction during a sterilization cycle. Manual cleaning of surgical instruments, glassware and other equipment is a time-consuming, sometimes hazardous and expensive burden for many institutions, particularly in the light of the increased number of operations performed in the past decade.

Within recent years manufacturers have developed equipment to overcome the problem. This equipment is called an ultrasonic cleaner or a sonic energy unit. This remarkable machine incorporates many major advances in electronic engineering. Electrical current is fed into an electronic generator, where it is converted into high frequency electrical energy. This energy, fed into "transducers," changes electrical energy to mechanical energy in the form of sound waves. These sound waves, passing through a solvent (volume of water and detergent), rapidly and thoroughly clean off soil from surfaces by a process called cavitation. The better ultrasonic cleaners incorporate a rinsing and a drying cycle.

Since these machines are cleaners and *not* sterilizers, personnel safety demands that instruments used in an operation be terminally sterilized in a pressure washer-sterilizer before being processed in a sonic energy unit.

CUTTING-EDGE INSTRUMENTS

The majority of sharp, cutting instruments such as general dissecting or suture scissors, osteotomes, chisels, and eyed suture needles are made of stainless steel and can be steam sterilized effectively within instrument sets.

A small number of cutting-edge instruments have a high carbon content in the steel and tend to dull, to corrode or to pit when steam sterilization methods are used. Delicate eye surgery instruments like keratomes and iris scissors are typical examples. With such instruments, then, other methods must be employed. When ethylene oxide or dry heat sterilization equipment is not available, disinfection of these instruments can be accomplished by a 3-hour period of submersion of the cleaned instruments in Bard-Parker Germicide or in Cidex. (Shorter periods of submersion

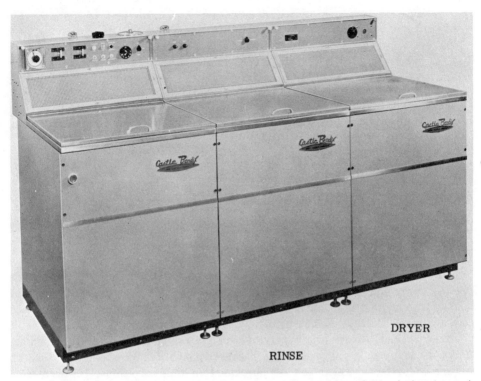

Fig. 23. Ultrasonic unit. Note 3-cabinet arrangement for washing (*left*), rinsing (*center*) and drying (*right*). (Wilmot Castle Company, Rochester, N.Y.)

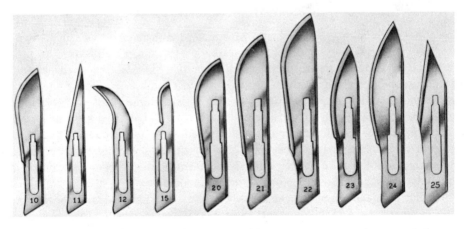

Fig. 24. The most common kinds of knife blades. (Becton, Dickinson and Company, Rutherford, N.J.)

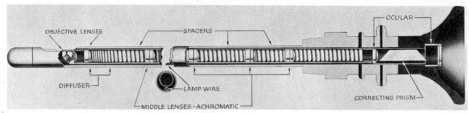

Fig. 25. Sectional view of typical telescope showing relation of parts in optical system. (American Cystoscope Makers, Inc., Pelham Manor, N.Y.)

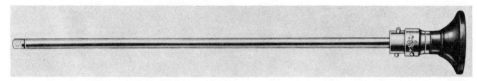

Fig. 26. Completed cystoscope. (American Cystoscope Makers, Inc.)

in aqueous "Quat" solutions kill only vegetative bacterial cells.) In the submerging process, care must be taken to avoid mechanical injury such as dulling an edge by contact with another instrument. Instruments soaked in any solution must be rinsed carefully in sterile distilled water before being used on a patient.

Knife (scalpel) blades in a variety of sizes are available from several manufacturers in wrapped, sterile, peelback packages. Such blades should be used in preference to those which can be purchased in bulk and must be disinfected chemically. Prewrapped sterile blades are available in carbon steel or in stainless steel. (Fig. 24)

ENDOSCOPY INSTRUMENTS

An endoscope is a long tubular instrument much like a telescope which is used to look within a body cavity. Some examples are a cystoscope, which is used to inspect the urinary bladder, a gastroscope, which is used to inspect the stomach, and a peritoneoscope, which is used to inspect the peritoneal cavity. These are optical instruments containing multiple small, precision-ground glass lenses. These instruments are equipped with light-carriers (attached to a battery box) to permit a distant image to be visualized through a long lumen (open tube).

Steam sterilization may *not* be used for instruments of this type, since high temperature and moisture tend to soften the cement holding the lenses, causing distortion of the image and making the instrument inoperable.

Alkaline germicides make the lens glass opaque, and some others (alcohol is one) may loosen the cement holding the lenses. Disinfection which provides tuberculocidal action can be achieved by a 10-minute submersion of the cleaned instruments in 10 per cent aqueous formalin or in activated glutaraldehyde (Cidex). Thorough rinsing in sterile distilled water is important before use on a patient. Ethylene oxide gas sterilization is the method of choice, although it may be necessary to return older instruments to the manufacturer for replacement of the cement with a type of adhesion that will tolerate this process. (Figs. 25, 26)

Fiber optics is a term used to describe a new type of illumination system for endoscopic instruments. This system replaces the conventional light-carrier, battery box and battery cable but utilizes present endoscopy equipment. A light-weight power supply box mounted 5 feet off the floor provides high intensity (rheostat-controlled) cool and constant light through a flexible cable (48 to 72 inches in length) of thin optical glass fibers. This major scientific achievement now permits concentration of high intensity light at the operative site without shadowing or diffusion. The connecting cables and fiber optics light-carriers may be disinfected as recommended for cystoscopes. However, the method of choice is to wrap the parts in polyethylene film and sterilize them with ethylene oxide gas. (Some fiber optics can be steam sterilized. See p. 114.) (Fig. 27)

SUTURE MATERIAL

A wide variety of threadlike material is used to sew tissues together (approximate) and to tie off (ligate) bleeding vessels. Suture materials used in modern hospitals are purchased from reliable manufacturers, and most of the sutures are in the form of packaged sterile units. The sterility of these sutures can be relied upon because of the rigid bacteriologic and other high-quality controls used by manufacturers.

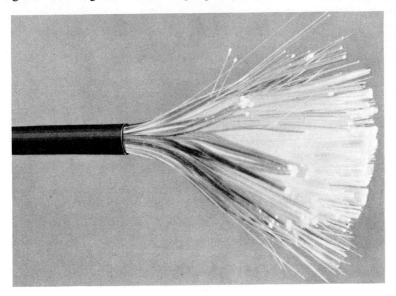

Fig. 27. A bundle of approximately 200,000 flexible optical fibers encased in a sturdy pliant cable. (American Cystoscope Makers, Inc.)

TYPES

Sutures are classified as absorbable or nonabsorbable. As these terms suggest, either the sutures will be absorbed by tissue fluids (or body enzymes) after 5 to 20 days, or they may remain within the body encapsulated as inert knots which usually cause no adverse reaction.

Absorbable suture material called *surgical gut* is available in a variety of sizes from 7-0 (very fine) to 3 (very heavy). There are two kinds of surgical gut, *plain* and *chromic*. Both of these kinds are prepared from the submucosa of sheep intestines. This particular intestinal layer is mechanically and chemically washed several times, split into ribbons and threads, stretched and cut into lengths, gauged, spun, polished, tested, packaged and sterilized. It is necessary to have some absorbable sutures which are more resistant to the enzyme action of tissue fluids so that they can support a healing wound for a longer period of time. To accomplish this, some strands of plain gut are treated with a chromium salt solution, which retards its absorption and digestion by body fluids. This additional step in the process of manufacture distinguishes chromic from plain surgical gut. Other less frequently used absorbable sutures are ribbon gut, fascia lata and kangaroo tendon.

Nonabsorbable Suture Material. The most widely used nonabsorbable suture material is *surgical silk*. The raw material comes from threads spun by silkworm larva in making their cocoons. Manufacturers then either twist the fibers or braid them in a variety of sizes ranging from 6-0 (very fine) to 4 (very heavy). Fine gauges of braided silk appear to be more popular because it is easier to handle than twisted silk. Silk sutures are made noncapillary (nonwicking) and serum-proof by impregnating them with wax, which remains through repeated sterilizations despite some loss in tensile strength. (Tensile strength is the amount of weight or pull necessary to break a knotted suture.) Silk sutures usually are dyed black for easy visibility in tissues. Some manufacturers use other colors to distinguish sizes.

Surgical cotton is a less frequently used nonabsorbable suture. It originates from cotton plants, and the fibers usually are twisted rather than braided. This suture generally is white, but some manufacturers have color-coded it according to the size of the strands. Cotton has the least tensile strength of all suture materials available, but it gains about 10 per cent in strength through sterilization. However, since it tends to shrink during steam sterilization, cut lengths should be prepared if nonsterile spools are used.

Other available types of nonabsorbable sutures include synthetic fibers of polyesters and nylon, dermal; metallic sutures of stainless steel, tantalum and silver; and metallic clips (used for clamping blood vessels in brain surgery).

SELECTION AND PREPARATION

In the selection and the use of suture materials the surgeon's preference is based on his experience and the needs of the patient. In most operating rooms flexible suture routines have been developed for each surgeon and each procedure.

Although most sutures are available in packaged, sterile units, some hospitals purchase silk, cotton and some metallic sutures on nonsterile spools. Before sterilizing these sutures, cut lengths or long strands should be removed from wooden spools to prevent chemical deposits in the wood from impregnating the sutures. Since sutures cost on an average of 45 cents per strand, care and economy must be exercised to avoid misuse and waste. Once opened, sutures should be handled as little as possible to prevent fraying of strands.

NEEDLES

SURGICAL NEEDLES

Many types of surgical needles are available, and their use and selection are based on the patient's needs and the surgeon's preference. There are regular-eyed needles with eyes that are round or square, shafts that are straight or curved, and points that are cutting, spear, tapering, trocar or blunt. Each of these is threaded much like a household sewing needle. Whatever suture material is requested, a double strand of the thread is present at the eye end of the needle. This double strand must be pulled through tissue. (Figs. 28 to 30)

French needles in a variety of sizes and shapes have a springlike eye that is threaded by a steady pull of the suture over the spring. Although French needles are easier to thread than the regular-eyed needles, a double strand of the material remains to be pulled through tissue.

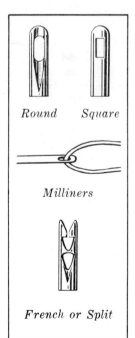

Round   Square

Milliners

French or Split

Fig. 28. Various types of eyed needles. (Davis & Geck, Division of American Cyanamid Company, Danbury, Conn.)

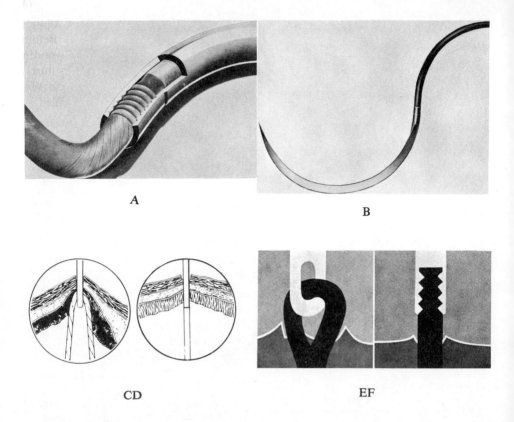

A

B

CD   EF

Fig. 29. (A) Cut view showing adherence of suture within needle. (B) Same diameter needle and suture. (C) Greater tissue trauma is caused by the double suture strand threaded through eyed needles. (D) Atraumatic needles cause minimum tissue trauma by eliminating the double suture strand. (E) Same as C. (F) Same as D. (A, E, F: Ethicon, Inc., Somerville, N.J.; B, C, D: Davis & Geck, Division of American Cyanamid Company, Danbury, Conn.)

Swaged needles, sometimes called atraumatic or Atraloc, reduce tissue trauma (injury), since the needles are permanently fused to the suture, leaving no eye to thread. This type of needle-suture combination is rapidly replacing eyed suture technics because of the many benefits to patients, surgeons and personnel.

OTHER NEEDLES USED IN SURGERY

Included in this list are hypodermic and intravenous needles, spinal needles, and cannulated needles used for neurosurgery and other services. To avoid the possible

BASIC SURGICAL NEEDLE COMPONENTS

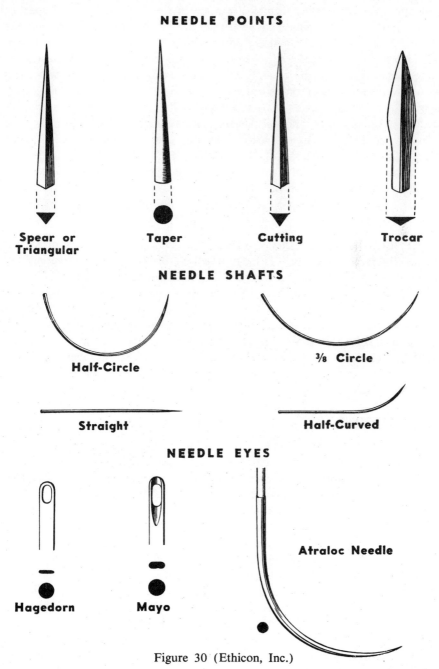

NEEDLE POINTS

Spear or Triangular
Taper
Cutting
Trocar

NEEDLE SHAFTS

Half-Circle
³⁄₈ Circle
Straight
Half-Curved

NEEDLE EYES

Hagedorn
Mayo
Atraloc Needle

Figure 30 (Ethicon, Inc.)

transmission of the hepatitis virus to personnel, used needles should be terminally processed in a pressure washer-sterilizer before definitive cleaning is done.

Cleaning and reprocessing usually are done in the Central Service Department either by hand or by machine. Soaked first in a mild detergent solution, the entire needle—the outside, the hub and the part within the tubular wall (lumen)—must be made scrupulously clean. After swabbing with cotton-tipped applicators and flushing each lumen with the pressure of a large syringe, multiple tap water rinses followed by distilled water rinses are necessary to remove all traces of detergent compound. Individual paper packages of cleaned needles usually are sterilized in an autoclave along with other packages going through a standard cycle. Since needles have lumens, it is important to moisten the lumen; the moisture will convert to steam and sterilize the interior of the needle.

Patient and personnel safety, as well as the cost of reprocessing needles, justifies the purchase and the use of sterile disposable needles.

GLASSWARE

Glassware used in surgery usually includes various sizes and types of syringes, medicine glasses and test tubes. After terminal sterilization in the operating room, these items generally are reprocessed in the Central Service Department. Here they are washed by hand or by machine. Care must be used in handling glassware to avoid cuts and breakage. Each article should be carefully rinsed free of detergent solution and then packaged. They may be either individually wrapped in paper or muslin or included within sets and sterilized in a standard steam cycle.

Sterile disposable syringes now are available and economically feasible for most hospitals. Medicine glasses should be replaced with metal cups, which are easier to clean and to handle.

SOLUTIONS

In most hospitals the preparation of solutions for external or internal use is done in the Central Service Department. These solutions generally include isotonic sodium chloride solution (normal saline, usually 0.9% C.P. salt in water), distilled water, glycine and other urologic solutions, and magnesium sulfate solution.

Although some hospitals buy commercially prepared solutions for external use, the vast majority of institutions purchase commercially prepared solutions, such as intravenous fluids, for use in parenteral routes. The reason is that pharmaceutical firms use chemically pure compounds and exercise rigid quality controls on each flask, assuring accuracy, stability, sterility and safety.

Hospital-made solutions for external use should be carefully controlled and prepared in a manner to meet the high standards set by firms making parenteral solutions. When solutions for external use are used to bathe tissues in irrigating a deep wound, the absorption qualities are similar to those of intravenous fluids. Solutions for external use are necessary in hospitals to wash and to rinse equipment and, when sterile, to bathe tissues, to irrigate cavities, to moisten sponges, and to rinse off instruments as well as gloved hands during an operative procedure.

There is scarcely a procedure involving patient care that does not require the use of water. As taken from a tap, depending on the locality, water is hard or soft. Hard water generally has a large amount of calcium, some magnesium and iron compounds. Soft water contains only small amounts of these chemicals. To remove them, water is distilled. Fluids for external use usually are prepared from distilled water, which is made in a water still. Distillation is a simple process of heating water until it boils and changes into steam vapor. When the steam is cooled, the vapor converts to water again, leaving in the vessel where the boiling took place the impurities that originally were in the water. These impurities include bacteria, pyrogens (toxic products of bacterial activity), minerals and soil.

To produce water of high purity, water stills are mandatory in a solution preparation program. Some stills manufactured today provide water of exceptional purity. However, in order to render this water sterile for use in an operating room, it is necessary to transfer the water from the reservoir into specially designed vacuum flasks which are made of heat-resistant glass such as Pyrex.

Flasks are available in a variety of sizes, equipped with collars and caps which can be vented during the sterilization cycle to provide a vacuum seal. Solution flasks are sterilized as separate loads in an autoclave. All sizes up to 1,000 cc. (1 qt.) are sterilized for 30 minutes at 250° F. Larger flasks are exposed for 45 minutes at 250° F. Following the appropriate sterilization cycle, the steam valve is turned to the "Off" position to allow the temperature to drop slowly. In some sterilizers a "Slow Exhaust" is used to evacuate the chamber steam. The use of "Fast Exhaust" (used for textiles) is avoided in solution sterilization, because rapid displacement of steam and reduction of temperature may cause explosive vaporization of solutions, resulting in blown-off caps and sometimes broken bottles. Manufacturers' recommendations should be followed in the care, the handling and the sterilization of solutions and flasks. Appropriate labels of metal or cardboard should be attached to each flask to indicate its contents. After the solutions have been sterilized and cooled at room temperature, a light blow on the top or the bottom of a flask with the heel of the hand should produce a distinctive click that is called "water hammer." If sterilization time and temperature have been adequate for the load, the "water hammer" indicates that a vacuum seal has been accomplished; the solutions then are safe for use immediately, or they may be stored indefinitely. (Figs. 32, 33)

A safe and convenient carrier for heated flasks is shown on page 108.

RUBBER GOODS

Rubber gloves, drains, catheters, tubing, and equipment for anesthesia machines also are handled by operating room personnel.

Care, handling, preparation and sterilization of rubber goods present some

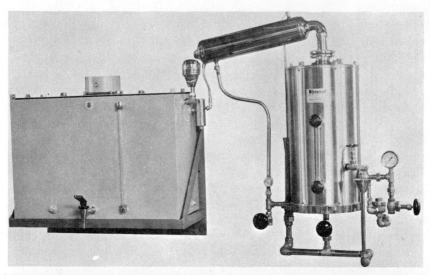

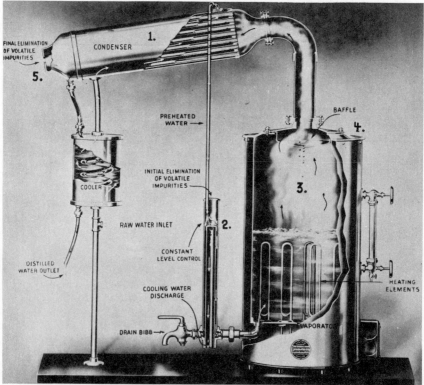

Fig. 31. (*Top*) Still and reservoir. (*Bottom*) How the Barnstead still operates. (Barnstead Still and Sterilizer Co., Boston, Mass.)

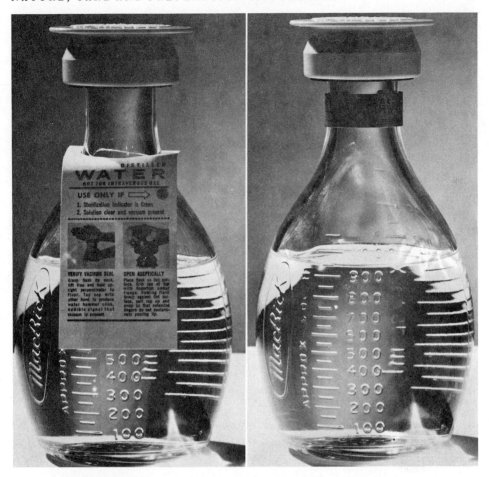

Fig. 32. Solution flasks. Flask on left demonstrates the new cardboard labeling technic which provides directions as well as visual identification. On right is the stainless steel metal neckband type of identification. (The Macbick Company, Wilmington, Mass.)

special problems. Natural rubber is of vegetable origin; heat, sunlight, grease, oils and solvents can destroy it readily. When any rubber material is intended for reuse, the prompt removal of deteriorating matter or conditions is important.

RUBBER GLOVES

Although disposable sterile rubber gloves are becoming increasingly popular, many hospitals continue to purchase rubber gloves for processing and reuse. Before new gloves are used, they should be washed to clean off talcum or other residue remaining on the rubber after the gloves were removed from the manufacturer's

A. INTERIOR COLLAR GROOVE EFFECTS AIR-TIGHT SEAL AGAINST BEADED LIP OF FLASKS.

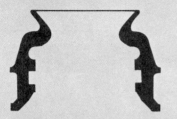

B. HOLDER LUGS GRASP COLLAR BEAD TO PREVENT POP-OFF OF HOOD.

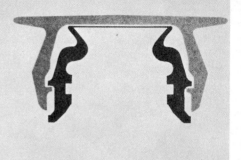

I. ASSEMBLY PROCEDURE:

1. Push collar down firmly onto neck of filled-flask so that groove inside collar securely grasps the heavy-beaded lip of the flask neck finish. (See A.)
2. Place hood squarely on rubber collar and push down gently so that all holder lugs on the inner surface of the hood snap under the bead on the collar exterior. (See B.) **Improper placement of hood may cause lip to depress irregularly causing failure of closure to seal under vacuum.**

II. STERILIZATION PROCEDURE:

1. Place capped flasks in autoclave. Admit steam to chamber and autoclave at 250°F (Exhaust line temperature) at 15 lbs. pressure for 30 continuous minutes.
2. Close steam valve when sterilization period is completed; allow chamber pressure to return to zero pounds pressure (usually requires 20-40 minutes for autoclave of up to 24″ x 36″ x 60″ size). As sterilizer pressure drops, pressure within flask is reduced by venting of steam through air vents (See C.). **Too rapid exhaust of autoclave pressure may cause hoods to "pop" off or may result in abnormal fluid loss.**
3. **Open chamber door slowly, and carefully withdraw the sterilizer car and carriage. Leave flasks undisturbed on sterilizer car until cool.** The closures "hum" as they exhaust steam from the flasks. When the pressure inside of the flask is relieved and equalizes with atmospheric pressure, the hoods seal against the collar lip. As the solutions cool and remaining steam within the flask condenses, the attendent vacuum pulls the hood firmly against the lip; the secondary seal is also achieved to complete the closure's hermetic seal of the flask.

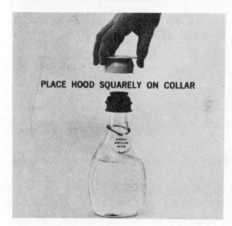

PLACE HOOD SQUARELY ON COLLAR

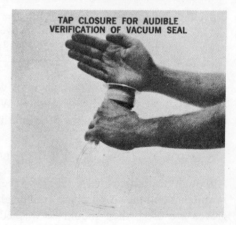

TAP CLOSURE FOR AUDIBLE VERIFICATION OF VACUUM SEAL

Fig. 33. Principles underlying vacuum seal. (The Macbick Company)

C. HOOD VENTS FLASK DURING COOL-DOWN PHASE OF STERILIZATION CYCLE.

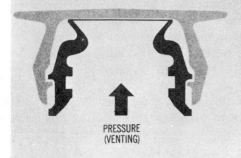

PRESSURE
(VENTING)

D. CONDENSING STEAM WITHIN COOLING FLASK CREATES VACUUM SEAL.

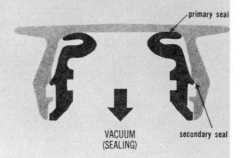

primary seal

VACUUM
(SEALING)

secondary seal

USE PROCEDURE:

1. Verify vacuum seal maintenance by gently jarring flask just prior to use. NOTE: The water-hammer click denotes that flask is vacuum sealed. Obviously a vacuum seal is necessary to maintain sterility once attained. The water hammer audible signal is a most desirable safety feature because it ascertains that the hermetic seal has not leaked during storage. **To jar the flask, grasp the neck with one hand, lift the flask free and hold it at a 45° angle with the closure facing you. Gently tap the hooded closure with the edge of the other hand.**
2. Heat flask to desired temperature* in solution warmers or solution warming cabinets. **Remove heated flask by means of the appropriate flask tong.**
3. Remove hood at sterile field. **Place the flask so that its base is firmly set onto a flat surface.** Grasp the neck with one hand and with the other hand grasp the hood so that the palm presses down on the top surface and so that the finger tips hook under and press up against the underside of the hood flange. As you **firmly hold the flask against the flat surface on which it is placed**, pull the hood toward you, up and away from the collar so that the sterile lip-shoulder area is not contaminated by extended finger tips.
4. Pour sterile contents into sterile solution basins.
5. Unused contents of the flask may be temporarily aseptically resealed by replacing the hood so as to protect the sterility of the lip-shoulder area. But such **unused contents must be discarded at the close of the case.**

IV. DISASSEMBLY PROCEDURE:

A. At Point of Use:
1. Discard unused contents of containers after surgical case is completed.
2. Replace hood as a dustproof seal for the empty container.
3. Return solutions unit to fluids preparation department at the close of the day.

B. At Preparation Department:
1. Remove hoods.
2. Remove collars. No tools are required. By grasping underside of skirt with fingers and lifting up while bearing down on distal lip with heel of hand, collar is easily removed. A point to remember is that wet closures are more easily placed on and removed from flasks — if difficulty is experienced in assembly or disassembly of components, wet the closure by submerging same under distilled water.
3. Clean-up procedure is then followed as outlined in Section I.

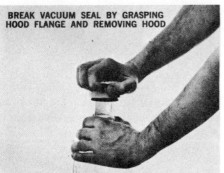

BREAK VACUUM SEAL BY GRASPING HOOD FLANGE AND REMOVING HOOD

*NOTE: DO NOT HEAT OTHER TYPES OF SOLUTION UNITS. SOFT GLASS BOTTLES, EQUIPPED WITH NON-VENTING SEALS, FOR EXAMPLE, MAY EXPLODE IF HEATED.

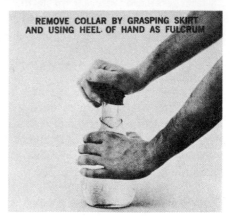

REMOVE COLLAR BY GRASPING SKIRT AND USING HEEL OF HAND AS FULCRUM

mold. Soaking new gloves for 15 minutes in a 5 per cent sodium carbonate solution followed by rinsing will remove what irritants remain on the rubber.

Immediately after each operation, to eliminate blood and debris, gloves should be washed off under cold water before removal from the hands. Throughout the day used gloves should be collected in a wide-mesh bag and sent preferably to the laundry or to Central Service for machine washing in a mild alkali detergent like Tide or Oakite. After the rinsing cycle the gloves can be dried in the laundry tumbler, which is set at its lowest temperature (around 120° F.). If this is not possible, in Central Service they should be placed in a glove drier. Next, they are placed in a glove powdering machine, where a cornstarch derivative powder is added to lubricate the rubber. After air-testing to eliminate those with holes, the gloves are sorted, paired and ready for packaging. In determining packaging procedure, it must be remembered that in steam sterilization of rubber gloves the problem is not steam penetration through many layers of material but rather effective air removal from the glove fingers. Wrapping of gloves must provide a means for exposing all surfaces to steam.

A single-thickness billfold type muslin wrapper (or a similar arrangement in quality paper) serves well as a protective cover. Wrapping this in a double-thickness muslin square or an effective single-thickness paper square secured with a small piece of tabbed autoclave tape completes the package.

Wrapped packages are placed in a rack with glove thumbs up, and the racks are located in the upper two thirds of the sterilizer chamber. During the cycle they almost immediately become enveloped in moisture, and this prevents the destructive effect of superheating. A safe minimum standard for sterilization of rubber goods is 20 minutes at 250° F. However, many hospitals effectively use the 30-minute standard exposure cycle for all goods. Drying within the chamber for 15 minutes with the door "cracked," followed by air drying at room temperature, will further avoid superheating. Longevity of rubber gloves is improved by a 48-hour rest period after steam sterilization.

Ethylene oxide sterilization is also effective for rubber gloves. A 24-hour aeration period is recommended to eliminate all absorbed gases.

DRAINS, CATHETERS, TUBING

These materials should be cleaned in an alkali detergent and thoroughly rinsed in tap water and then in distilled water. Immediately before packaging them in muslin or paper wrappers, moisture should be flushed through the lumens to permit sterilization of the interior of the tubes.

Many types of sterile disposable catheters, drains and tubing are available and are in use in several hospitals.

ANESTHESIA MACHINE EQUIPMENT

The care and the processing of rubber parts of anesthesia machines, i.e., face masks, rebreathing bags, corrugated hoses and endotracheal tubes, are the responsibility of the personnel on the anesthesia service. A large enough inventory of parts should be available to permit the technics of adequate cleaning, disinfecting and, ideally, sterilizing them between patients. Immediately after use the parts can be submerged in a detergent-germicidal solution of a synthetic phenolic or iodine for 15 minutes. This is followed by manual cleaning of parts in a similar solution. Careful rinsing in copious amounts of water will remove all chemical residue. The ideal then is to place the parts within a thin polyethylene bag and to sterilize them in ethylene oxide. A 24-hour aeration period will eliminate the absorbed gases.

PLASTIC MATERIALS

Self-adhering disposable surgical drapes are perhaps the most popular of plastic materials used in operating rooms. These products pose no problems in processing, because they are packaged and sterilized by the manufacturers. This is true also of plastic disposable syringes.

There are a variety of plastic tubings available, many of which can be steam sterilized. However, polyethylene tubing may melt in autoclaving. If ethylene oxide is not available, such material must be disinfected chemically as described on pages 59 and 60.

Other nonheat-stable plastic materials should be sterilized in ethylene oxide. If this is not possible, chemical disinfection methods must be employed.

ELECTRICAL EQUIPMENT

Electric bone-saws, electric dermatomes, electric dental drills, cautery cords, etc., should be wrapped and kept sterile for emergency use. Packaged in muslin or paper, they may be steam sterilized with instrument sets or wrapped individually for sterilization. After the goods have cooled and dried, the unit may be placed in a clean polyethylene bag, which is sealed. In this manner an indefinite period of sterile storage can be attained.

The electric motors in these devices probably will last longer if they are sterilized by ethylene oxide rather than by steam. When the former method is employed, paper wrapping plus polyethylene film wrapping can secure the article and, after sterilization and a 24-hour aeration period, protect the sterile packages for an indefinite shelf-life.

RADIUM AND RADIOISOTOPES

Establishment of specific hospital policies designed to protect patients and personnel and to control radiation is mandatory for all hospitals using this type of therapy.

Control of radium and radon is usually the responsibility of the hospital's radiologist, who maintains a remote lead-lined vault for storage of these materials. X-ray personnel should be taught safe methods of handling the materials and the need for lead shielding during the mounting of various tampons or filling needles with radon seeds. The equipment to be used on patients is transported in alcohol solution in a thick lead carrier, and thus it is brought into the operating room. This carrier remains closed until the surgeon has need for the material.

Radioisotopes usually are controlled by the hospital's pathologist. Patients undergoing diagnostic procedures are no threat to personnel. However, patients given therapeutic doses are treated with the same precautions as are radium patients.

Hospital policies should carefully define the need for film badges, lead shields and aprons, visual aids denoting radiation areas, special precautions regarding handling and transporting, and the significance of the length of exposure and distance from the source.

LENGTH OF TIME SUPPLIES REMAIN STERILE

An apparent controversy exists on this subject. Some hospitals rewrap and resterilize packages every week or every 2 weeks. The studies done on this subject are scanty, but the latest data indicates that supplies wrapped in either muslin or special paper remain sterile for at least 4 weeks. These studies presuppose that the wrappers are good protective covers, that the storage areas are clean and free from flying or crawling insects, and that atmospheric conditions remain relatively constant.

In a well organized and managed operating room or Central Service, it is reasonable to assume that inventory levels of supplies would be geared to a turnover of sterile goods within 1 month. Therefore, excessive inventory levels cause unnecessary work for many personnel. At any rate, in modern hospitals there is no need to resterilize goods every week or every 2 weeks.

SUMMARY

In summary, there are a variety of materials which are used in hospitals. With the many methods of sterilization available, the safest, fastest and least expensive method is saturated steam under pressure. Where this method will not destroy the particular article, it is the method of choice. Other methods of sterilization and/or disinfection also are important and are based on sound scientific principles. With a clear understanding of the methods of cleaning, handling and packaging of supplies, sterilization procedures will be safe and successful.

REVIEW QUESTIONS:
1. What is meant by "terminal sterilization" of instruments?
2. What does a sonic energy unit accomplish?
3. Why is chemical disinfection used for processing sharp instruments when steam is a more effective method?

4. Why do endoscopy instruments require special handling?
5. What are the differences between absorbable and nonabsorbable sutures?
6. What makes swaged-needled sutures more desirable than other types of sutures?
7. What makes distilled water more desirable for surgical procedures than tap water?
8. What does a "water hammer" sound signify?
9. What factors cause deterioration of rubber goods?
10. What factors contribute to the length of time goods remain sterile?

Bibliography

Perkins, J. J.: Principles and Methods of Sterilization, Springfield, Ill., Thomas, 1956.
Walter, C. W.: The Aseptic Treatment of Wounds, New York, Macmillan, 1948.

CHAPTER 6

PREPARATION AND SPECIFIC RESPONSIBILITIES OF OPERATING ROOM PERSONNEL

CLASSIFICATION : GENERAL PREPARATION : SKIN ANTISEPSIS :

GOWNING : GLOVING : RESPONSIBILITIES OF THE CIRCULATING

NURSE : HANDLING OF STERILE SUPPLIES AND EQUIPMENT IN

THE OPERATING ROOM

CLASSIFICATION

Operating room nursing personnel have been described and categorized as professional and nonprofessional workers (Chaps. 1 and 2). Personnel are classified also according to the function performed as a member of the surgical team. Hence, the worker may be scrubbed ("sterile") or unscrubbed ("unsterile"). When scrubbed, the professional nurse is commonly referred to as the "scrub nurse" or "suture nurse." Should her responsibilities be limited to the handling of sponges, she may be called a "sponge nurse." When scrubbed, the operating room technician usually is referred to as the "scrubbed nursing assistant," "scrubbed assistant," and even "scrub assistant." The scrub nurse or the scrubbed nursing assistant performs the duties described in this crapter in the sections on scrubbing, gowning, gloving and handling of sterile supplies and equipment.

The professional nurse who is not scrubbed but performs as the person supervising the activities within the particular operating room, and who also acts as coordinator and teacher of students and technicians, is referred to as the "circulating nurse" or the "circulator." She is a well-prepared professional nurse whose function is described in greater detail on page 96. The surgical technician may act as an "assistant circulator" to the professional nurse. Legally, however, the technician is neither expected nor prepared to act as the circulating (charge) nurse.

GENERAL PREPARATION

Operating room personnel are concerned with protecting the patient from pain, hemorrhage and infection. The problem of pain is handled by the anesthesia department; the control of hemorrhage is managed by the surgeon, who has various means at his disposal; however, the problem of infection must be the responsibility of *everyone* who enters the operating room. Moisture droplets or dust can carry infection from several sources into a wound. Such contamination can come from air entering the room, from the exhalations of personnel, from the hands and the clothing of personnel and from the patient's own skin and body. This section will be concerned with the precautions each member of the operating team can take to insure maximum protection of the patient from infection.

Personal Hygiene

Everyone who enters the operating floor must be clean and healthy. Personal hygiene includes (1) a daily bath, (2) skin in good condition (free from cuts or lesions, particularly if one scrubs for an operation), and (3) hair that is clean, controlled and as free from dust and dandruff particles as possible. Nails should be well trimmed and clean. An upper respiratory infection in any person in the operating room can be a source of infection to a patient; since the nose and the mouth are sources of bacteria, it is desirable to limit conversation, sneezing, coughing and laughing. Being in a state of general good health permits a worker to perform at his optimum level; hence adequate nutrition, sufficient rest and sleep, time for recreation as well as the avoidance of undue fatigue are essential requirements. Persistent use of alcohol or medications which dull the thinking processes also is not helpful for the person who needs to be alert and quick-thinking at all times.

Clothing and Shoes

No article of outer clothing, including shoes which have been worn in the street or in other parts of the hospital, should be worn in the operating room. Likewise, streetwear should not hang near operating room clothing.

Women wear short-sleeved cotton dresses of simple design, with the sleeves at least 3 inches above the elbow. A tie belt is used to keep the dress close to the body, thereby preventing it from touching a sterile area. Men wear short-sleeved cotton top shirts and trousers which have drawstrings to secure the trousers at the waist over the shirt. Soft blue or green is preferred to white because it is easier on the eyes. These outfits are changed daily or more often if necessary. Silk, wool, nylon, dacron and other synthetic textile materials are not worn in the operating or anesthetizing rooms because of the danger of causing static electrical sparks when two such surfaces rub together. This would be an explosive hazard because of the possibility of electrostatic energy buildup in the presence of inflammable anesthetic gases. (Nylon stockings or underwear worn close to the body are permissible.)

If the operating room floor has electrically conductive flooring, as it should, conductive shoes should be worn. The purpose of this system is to drain off accumulated static electricity harmlessly into the ground. To ensure proper grounding, conductivity of the shoes should be checked with a conductivity meter. In the case of visitors, a disposable conductive shoe covering usually is provided. Shoes should be kept clean not only for the sake of appearance but also because they can be a place where dirt collects and organisms grow. Blood and soil must be scrubbed off mechanically with a soap solution, detergent or disinfectant, and each shoe must be cleaned daily. When footwear is clean and its use limited to the operating room, and when a satisfactory program of floor sanitization is carried out daily, potent sources of bacterial contamination are reduced.

Hair

Hair usually is contained in a cotton or disposable paper cap, with tie strings in the back for men and a turban or a helmet of cotton or disposable paper for women. The objective is to keep all hair covered, since it may be a source of sparks or contamination. Head covers are put on fresh and clean each day. It is recommended that the cap be put on before the dress or suit. If the dress is put on first, it is common practice for the person to comb his hair before putting on the cap. Hairs can fall on the shoulder of the dress and present a source of contamination.

Mask

The nose and the mouth of each person must be covered with a mask before entering the operating room. Ideally, a mask should be effective in filtering organisms of exhalation, thereby restricting their invasion of the atmosphere, and yet the mask should be comfortable to the wearer, allowing him to breathe easily. There are many kinds of masks on the market, with each company professing its mask to be the best. (Fig. 34)

To be effective, a mask should be worn snugly; if worn loosely, expired air escapes around the edges into the room. A moist mask becomes a poor filter, allowing organisms to pass around the sides rather than through it. This means that, to be effective, a wet or moist mask must be replaced by a dry one. Talking,

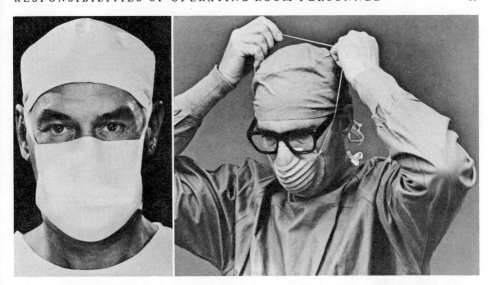

Fig. 34. (*Left*) Bardic deseret filtermask. (C. R. Bard, Inc., Murray Hill, N.J.) (*Right*) Disposable mask. (Minnesota Mining and Manufacturing Company, St. Paul, Minn.)

sneezing or coughing into a mask increases the bacteria forced into the air; such forced expiration should be avoided.

For those who wear glasses, fogging may be a problem while a mask is worn. To prevent glass surfaces from steaming, rub them with a piece of soap, soap powder or detergent. A malleable metal strip or contour-fitting section over the bridge of the nose also will prevent glasses from steaming.

SKIN ANTISEPSIS

THE NATURE OF SKIN

In order to understand the reason that certain methods of scrubbing are preferred over others, it becomes necessary to know the nature of skin. Skin is a soft flexible envelope covering the body completely, and at the natural orifices it is continuous with the mucous membranes. The skin is made up of two layers (Fig. 35): (1) the epidermis or surface layer and (2) the dermis (corium) or true skin. The epidermis is constantly being rubbed off and replaced with newly formed tissue. On some parts of the body where there is greater friction, such as the palm of the hand, the elbow, etc., this layer is thicker than on other parts. The dermis contains many sebaceous and sweat glands, blood vessels, nerves and roots of the hairs. Sebaceous glands secrete oil (sebum), which is mixed with dirt and bacteria. Sweat glands, which are especially numerous on the palms, secrete fatty and odorous substances as well as sweat. The complex structure of the skin is such that the many tiny openings on the skin make it extremely difficult to clean and impossible to sterilize. The bacterial flora found on the skin is classified in two groups: (1) transient and (2) resident. Transient flora are acquired by contact and are only loosely attached to the skin surface, but they may contain pathogenic organisms. Resident flora are found below the skin surface and are embedded in the crevices of the skin and in the sebaceous glands. (Fig. 35)

SCRUBBING

Since skin sterilization is impossible, the next best thing is to reduce the bacterial count of the skin to levels considered to be safe for surgery, a statement that is true for the operative site of the patient as well as the hands of the members of the operating team. This can be accomplished by scrubbing mechanically and using chemical antisepsis.

Hexachlorophene (G-11), a white powdered chemical related in chemical structure to the phenols, increases the bactericidal efficiency when added to certain

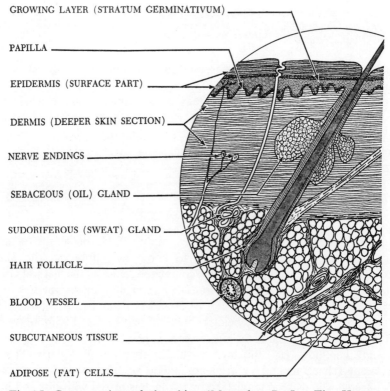

GROWING LAYER (STRATUM GERMINATIVUM)

PAPILLA

EPIDERMIS (SURFACE PART)

DERMIS (DEEPER SKIN SECTION)

NERVE ENDINGS

SEBACEOUS (OIL) GLAND

SUDORIFEROUS (SWEAT) GLAND

HAIR FOLLICLE

BLOOD VESSEL

SUBCUTANEOUS TISSUE

ADIPOSE (FAT) CELLS

Fig. 35. Cross section of the skin. (Memmler, R. L.: The Human Body in Health and Disease, ed. 2, p. 207, Philadelphia, Lippincott, 1962)

other preparations. Furthermore, hexachlorophene has the property of coating the skin with a filmy layer of the chemical that prolongs its action against resident bacteria. Because of the cumulative and continuing effectiveness of G-11, additional scrubs on the same day do not require as much time as the initial scrub, provided that the individual has been scrubbing the previous several days.

Scrubbing procedures should be standardized and followed by all without exception.

1. Nails should be short (not only to facilitate cleaning but also to prevent glove damage), and fingers must be free of hangnails. Nail polish of the chipping variety should be avoided.

2. Special attention should be given to the area under the nail (subungual area). This can be accomplished by using a sterile stainless steel nail file during the scrub.

3. Use a sterile brush, preferably one of nylon that is dispensed from a sterile covered container.

4. A definite pattern of strokes should be followed conscientiously as the individual scrubs each finger, the hand and then the arm, so that no area is inadvertently overlooked.

5. Hands always are held above the level of the elbow, so that contaminated drippings can roll off at the elbow. Otherwise, such drippings would run down to the hands and the fingers, the area that one is attempting to clean thoroughly.

Rockwell[1] describes a long scrub for the first of the day and a short scrub for use between cases.

THE LONG SCRUB

1. Wash hands and arms well with detergent agent. This is to get the skin surfaces wet and to remove the gross dirt before taking the brush.

2. Scrub with brush and agent using the following number of strokes. Hands: 20 strokes to nails; 10 strokes to surfaces of fingers and hands. Arms: 6 strokes to surfaces of arms to well above elbows. Add sufficient amounts of soap and water to maintain good lather.

3. Rinse: fingertips first, then hand, arm and elbow. Transfer brush to other hand.

4. Scrub the other hand and arm in the above manner.

5. Rinse. Discard brush in receptacle.

6. Clean subungual spaces with nail file or orangewood stick under running water.

7. Take clean brush, repeat above scrub procedure, substituting the following stroke count for both hands. Hands: 10 strokes to nails; 6 strokes to surfaces of fingers and hands. Arms: 3 strokes to arms to just below elbows.

8. Rinse well, fingertips to elbows, and discard brush.

9. Hold hands up with arms well away from body and proceed to operating room.

---

[1] Rockwell, V. A.: Surgical hand-scrubbing, Am. J. Nurs. 63:75–81, June 1963.

THE SHORT SCRUB

1. Wash hands and arms well.
2. Clean nails, with file or orangewood stick, under running water.
3. Scrub with brush: one hand and arm and then the other hand and arm, using the following brush stroke count: Hands: 20 strokes to nails; 10 strokes to fingers and surfaces of hands. Arms: 6 strokes to below elbows.
4. Rinse hands and arms. Discard brush.

Immediately following the scrub, the hands and the forearms must be held higher than the elbows so that water will drip off the elbows and not run down the arms to contaminate the hands.

ARM RINSE OR DIP

Authorities agree that a postscrub rinse is justified for two reasons. One is that many resident bacteria remain after scrubbing, and the other is that bacteria continue to grow and to multiply under rubber gloves. An arm rinse in a germicide solution helps to reduce these problems. The community basin or dip commonly is used for this purpose, but with repeated dippings the concentration of the solution is affected. The disadvantages of the basin hand dip can be minimized if each person dries his hands well before immersing them in the basin. (Water that would have been on the hands and the arms would increase the dilution of the solution.) Most hospitals which use "Quats" have changed the concentration from 1:1000 (an active germicide at this dilution) to 1:750 to provide a wider margin of safety. Other solutions which are being used are 95 per cent ethyl alcohol followed by a wash in 70 per cent ethyl alcohol; iodine solutions, such as 1 per cent iodine in 70 per cent alcohol; or PVP-I, iodine combined with PVP (polyvinylpyrrolidone), and a variety of others. It must be emphasized that the alcohol nullifies the action of hexachlorophene unless a compound of several alcohols which include hexachlorophene is used in the rinse. Some solutions require both washing and the application of friction, which enhance their effectiveness. Each hospital infection control committee should determine what cleansing agents are to be selected. Desirable characteristics are: effectiveness as a germicide; low surface tension, which permits maximum contact with skin surfaces; nonirritating effect; and that they be inexpensive and capable of prolonged bactericidal action.

A better method than the community basin is a dispenser which expresses individual quantities of germicide.

DRYING THE HANDS AND THE FOREARMS

Well-dried hands reduce the possibility of contamination and permit gloves to be donned more easily. Wet hands and arms would moisten the sterile gown, presenting a pathway for organisms to contaminate it from the unsterile scrub garb.

Drying of hands and arms must be done carefully and thoughtfully. The procedure is to grasp a folded sterile towel with one hand, permit it to unfold and hang to its full length. Then support the towel with both hands at the top, one on either side. Bending at the waist (Fig. 36) will prevent contamination of the lower end of the towel against the body. The fingers and hand of one arm are dried, and by rotating the wrist upward, the wrist and arm are dried to the elbow. The dried hand then grasps the free hanging portion of the towel, and the other hand and arm are dried in similar fashion. Care is taken so that no portion of the towel touching the skin of one hand or arm touches the other hand or arm. Then the towel is discarded.

Mechanical dryers with ultraviolet coils are effective and should be used where they are available. The nozzle is directed upward to allow bacteria-free warm air to dry the extended hands and arms. This system is desirable, since it avoids chapping of the skin.

GOWNING

The sterile gown may be obtained from an open pack, or it may be handed by someone already scrubbed. The gown is to be held at arm's length so that when it is unrolled, it will not touch one's suit or dress or any nearby objects. (A gown is folded in such a way that the inside faces outward, and the collar band can be

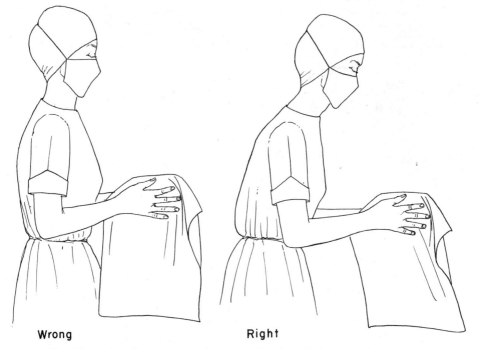

Wrong   Right

Fig. 36. By bending at the waist contamination of the towel is prevented.

grasped first. This is done to facilitate donning without touching the outside.) By holding the neckband, the gown can fall as it unrolls. By gently shaking the folds from the gown, the inside should face the wearer. The hands can be slipped into the armholes while the hands are held upward.

At this time the circulating nurse (see pp. 96, 97) reaches inside the gown to grasp the sleeve seam. By gently pulling she can pull the gown over the hands of the scrubbed person. Tapes at the back are tied. The circulating nurse reaches for the ends of the waist ties; the scrub nurse can lean slightly forward to swing the ties free from the gown. These are tied at the back. There are other kinds of gowns, but the principles remain the same.

GLOVING

OPEN METHOD

Before gloves are put on, the application of a glove lubricant to the hands will allow the hands to glide more easily into the gloves. Starch has largely replaced talcum inasmuch as the latter can cause adhesions in wounds due to chemical irritation and foreign body reaction. Nevertheless, powder contamination of the operative field still must be minimized. The use of commercially prepared lubricating cream is recommended. In some institutions adequate drying of the hands and the powder in the gloves are considered to be sufficient lubrication.

Gloves are packaged with a cuff of at least 2 inches. The objective is to put on the gloves without touching the outside of the glove or the gown with the bare hands.

In putting on the right glove, grasp its cuff on the *inside* with the left hand, insert the right hand into the glove and pull it in place with the left hand. Leave the cuff turned and release the grasp. Now the right gloved hand can pick up the left glove by inserting the fingers under its cuff (the outside is the sterile side). Insert the left hand in the left glove and pull into place leaving the cuff turned. By folding the gown wristlet snugly and holding this fold in place with the thumb of the opposite hand, that hand's fingers can safely pull up the

KEY POINTS
Keep arms at waist level or above.
Powder gently to minimize dust particles in the air.
Stand away from table when putting on gloves.
The skin of the hand can touch only the inside of the glove.
The outside of one glove can touch the outside of the other glove.

rubber glove cuff over the gown wristlet. Repeat for the other glove. (Fig. 37)

Offering the Gown and Gloves to One Who Has Just Scrubbed. In some hospitals it is the practice for a scrubbed person to hold the sterile gown and gloves for the surgeon in such a way that he is able to get into them easily. The following procedure is followed:

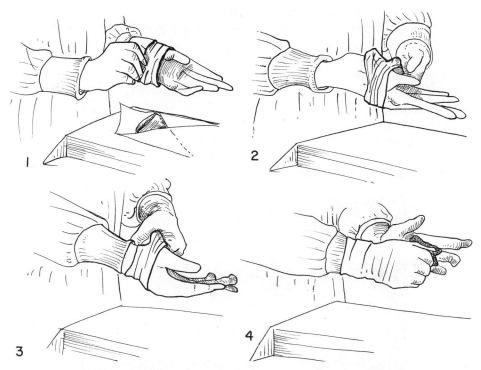

Fig. 37. (1) Pulling on left glove without touching outside. (2) Pulling on right glove by inserting gloved fingers into cuff. (3) Folding glove cuff over gown cuff. (4) Working on glove fingers with sterile gauze. (Redrawn from Brunner, L. S., *et al.*: Textbook of Medical-Surgical Nursing, pp. 240, 241, Figs. 51, 52, Philadelphia, Lippincott, 1964)

Gown. The scrub nurse holds out the rolled gown, grasps the neckband and lets the gown unfold. With the outside of the gown toward her, she makes a cuff at the neckband which covers her gloved hands. The inside of the gown is offered to the surgeon, who is facing her; meanwhile, the circulating nurse pulls the gown on and ties it.

Gloves. If a lubricant is used, the scrub nurse expresses the packet into the surgeon's hands or passes him the packet. She then cuffs and stretches the glove open in such a way that the thumb faces the surgeon (Fig. 38), and the inner side of the glove is the only part which he will touch as he slips his hand well into the glove. The scrub nurse pulls the cuff of the glove well over the surgeon's gown cuff.

CLOSED METHOD

Closed gloving technic provides a means of putting on sterile gown and gloves without the outside of the gown or gloves touching the skin. After scrubbing, the hands and the arms are pushed through the sterile gown up to the stockinette cuff.

The sleeve cuff seam is grasped, and the hands are not permitted to proceed outward through the cuff (Fig. 39A). Pick up the sterile (left) glove (Fig. 39B) and place it on the left arm of the gown, with the fingers pointing toward the shoulder, the thumb downward and the cuff touching the upper stockinette cuff edge. The opposite (right) sleeve-covered fingers grasp the upper glove cuff, and spread it apart (Fig. 39C) before pulling it down over the stockinette cuff (Fig. 39D), completely enclosing it (Fig. 39E). The opposite (right) sleeve-covered fingers then grasp both left gown and glove cuff and pull them on (Fig. 39F). The gloved hand repeats the procedure for putting on the other glove (Fig. 39G, H).

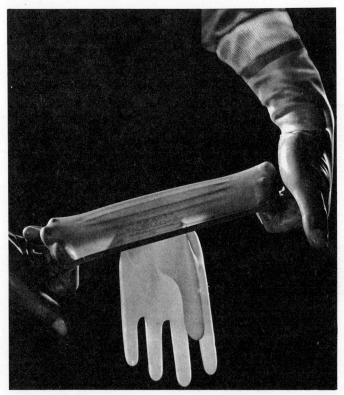

Fig. 38. The glove cuff is spread wide to allow the donner to slip his hand into the glove without touching the holder of the glove. Note that the thumb is facing toward the person who will wear the glove. (The Pioneer Rubber Company, Willard, Ohio)

RESPONSIBILITIES OF THE CIRCULATING NURSE

The circulating nurse (also called the circulator) is not scrubbed but is free to move about as she assists all other personnel before, during and after each operation. She is the key person in the proper and efficient management of all activities in the operating room. Because of her unique role, the circulator usually is a professional nurse. Briefly, her duties include the following categories. She

1. Greets, identifies, comforts and "oversees" the patient.

2. Understands principles of asepsis and their application.

3. Knows the care, sterilization, location and use of instruments, sutures, packs, and all other supplies used in an operating room.

4. Knows the care and safe operation of equipment such as surgical diathermy unit (Chap. 10), cautery, monitoring devices, and other special equipment.

5. Is familiar with preferences of the operating surgeon.

6. Has the ability to anticipate needs, such as the adjustment of lights, the need for more sponges, sutures, etc.

7. Is aware of the experience level and limitations of nursing and auxiliary personnel.

8. Understands and applies sound teaching and learning principles.

9. Understands and practices safety measures to prevent explosions or injury to patients and personnel.

10. Knows what procedure to follow in the event of an emergency such as cardiac arrest, power failure, etc.

11. Is familiar with hospital policy and regulations in matters that pertain to the operating room.

12. Can recognize and correct technic breaks.

13. Is skilled in interpersonal relations.

14. Understands the meaning of each operative procedure.

Additional responsibilities of the circulating nurse in preparing the operating room for the patient are discussed in Chapter 7, page 119. (Also see Fig. 40.) Those activities performed during the operative procedure are found in Chapter 10, page 191.

HANDLING OF STERILE SUPPLIES AND EQUIPMENT IN THE OPERATING ROOM

Sterile supplies needed by the operating team to perform the required surgery include linens, instruments, dressings, suture materials, needles, solutions, etc. The areas in which these supplies are assembled and used must be sterile. Hence, tables as well as the patient are covered with sterile drapes. These covers or sheets may be made of linen (cotton muslin fabric), plastic material or specially prepared waterproof paper.

Drapes and Draping

The effectiveness of drapes is determined by the extent of the barrier created against bacterial migration. Moisture is the means by which this movement of bacteria takes place when textile drapes are used. Therefore, it is preferred that

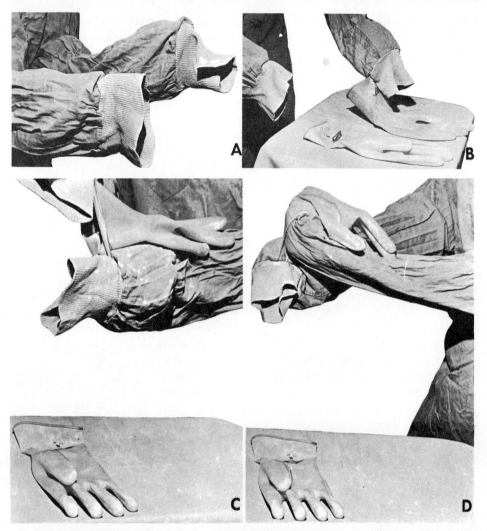

Fig. 39. Closed gloving technic. (The Pioneer Rubber Company, Willard, Ohio)

plastic or special waterproof paper be used. The latter has the additional advantages of being disposable, economical and lint-free.

When textile drapes are used, they should be hemmed or have selvage edges. For patient draping, such sheets should be of double thickness with reinforced thickness around the operative area and should be large enough to provide sufficient protection. Green, blue or gray are preferable to white drapes inasmuch as color reduces glare and eye fatigue. Green is credited with the advantage of providing contrast for color photography and television.

When the self-adhering drape is used, it is necessary that the operative site be thoroughly cleaned and dried before applying the plastic. The selection of such a

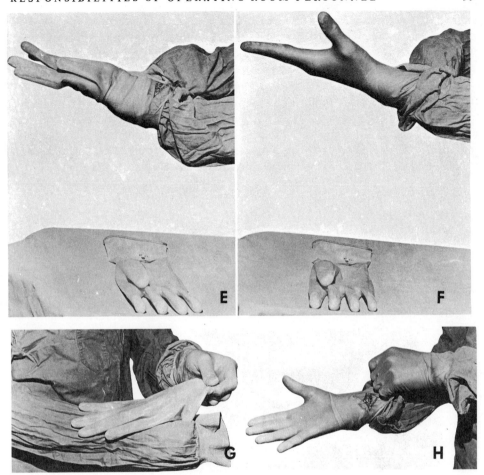

drape should include an evaluation of its electric spark potential. When antiseptics are used before the drape is applied, an interval of time must pass to insure thorough drying of the skin. The transparent plastic cover then is applied carefully; one member of the team spreads and smooths the drape from the incision site to the periphery to remove air bubbles and wrinkles (Fig. 41). Such a drape seals the skin and prevents wound contamination. It eliminates the need for towels and towel clips.

Regardless of the kind of material from which the drape is made, the principles of handling remain the same.

Folding of Drapes or Sheets.

1. *The drape is folded before sterilization in such a way that it can be handled easily and safely after sterilization.*

When the drape is used, it already is folded to insure keeping the upper side sterile. As it is placed on the table or the patient, the underside will become contaminated. Careful and safe handling of the drape is made easier by the use of a cuff, a turned down corner or by fanfolding or rolling. With these kinds of folds, the draper can protect her sterile gloved hands and the upper outer surface of the sheet as she unfolds it and places it where it is required.

2. *Sheets are folded to allow for easy and complete penetration of steam to all its surfaces during sterilization.*

This requirement can be demonstrated if one visualizes how a man's handkerchief is folded. If the handkerchief were made of plastic material, it would be impossible for steam to reach the innermost folds. However, if the handkerchief were fanfolded, all surfaces would be accessible. (See Packaging, p. 55.)

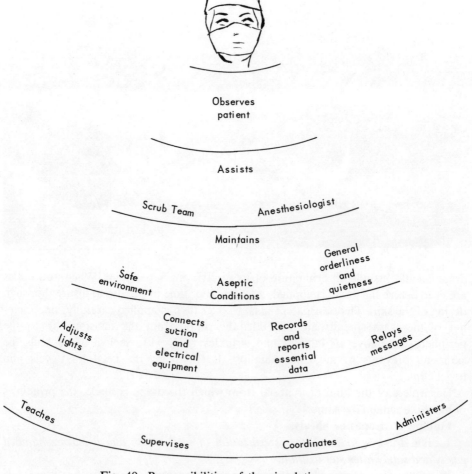

Fig. 40. Responsibilities of the circulating nurse.

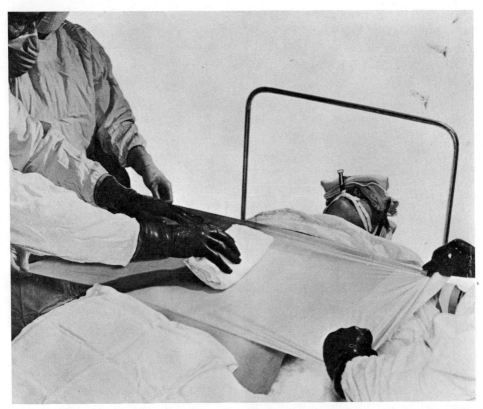

Fig. 41. Applying a plastic drape. Note that the surgeon is using a towel to press the drape to the incision site. By gently pressing the drape to the periphery, air bubbles and wrinkles will be eliminated. (Minnesota Mining and Manufacturing Company, St. Paul, Minn.)

GUIDE TO THE HANDLING OF STERILE DRAPES

Activity	*Principle*
Handle drapes as little as possible. Avoid shaking and flourishing of linens. Allow plenty of room to unfold drapes.	Air currents are capable of carrying contaminants.
Make a cuff or turn the corners of the drape over the gloved hand in preparation for spreading the drape and placing it on the patient or table with only the under surface of the drape touching the table or the patient.	Contact with an unsterile surface contaminates a sterile object.

Activity	*Principle*
In draping a table, the sheet is placed from the front to the back. Otherwise the front of the gown may touch the unsterile table.	Contact with an unsterile surface contaminates a sterile object.
Drapes should not be held so high that they touch the lights or other fixtures, or so low that they touch lower parts of furniture.	Contact with an unsterile surface contaminates a sterile object.
That part of the drape which falls below the top level of the table or the patient is considered to be unsafe as a sterile area.	When a question exists regarding the sterility of an area, the object (or field) is considered to be unsterile.
Drapes that have holes, tears or worn spots should not be used.	A portal of entry that allows contact with an unsterile surface immediately renders an otherwise sterile field contaminated.

Draping the Mayo Instrument Stand. This portable stand is a table that is placed above and across the feet of the patient to serve as a convenient area near the operative field for instruments that are constantly used.

The drape for such a stand is like a pillowcase. A cuff is made to protect the scrubbed person's hands. The balance of the drape is gathered and supported on the arms (never under the arms) to prevent its falling below waist-level. The Mayo stand can be stabilized by placing a foot on the base. Usually a snugly draped sterile tray is placed on top of the Mayo frame. (Fig. 42)

USE OF TRANSFER OR PICKUP FORCEPS

At times the scrub nurse needs a sterile object which may be located on another sterile table, in the autoclave or in a stock receptacle. This sterile object is transferred by the circulator, who uses a sterile pickup or transfer forceps. Such a forceps and its container are first sterilized (a single forceps for each container); then a germicide is added to the container, and the forceps is placed so that the prongs or the legs are immersed. Thereafter, only that end of the forceps which is in the germicide is considered to be sterile.

The forceps illustrated in Figure 43 automatically eliminates many of the possible sources of contamination and is highly recommended. The pistol grip permits comfortable handling; the bend in the instrument eliminates the need for consciously keeping the prongs pointed downward; and the type of prong permits the grasping of circular objects as well as fine surgical needles. The collar serves as a cap for the germicide container, thereby controlling unnecessary evaporation. A springlike guard within the container eliminates the problem of having the forceps touch the side above the solution level. As was stated in chemical dis-

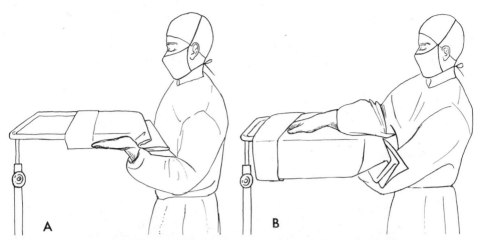

A   B

Fig. 42. (A) As the scrub assistant prepares to drape the Mayo stand, note that a cuff of linen protects his hands, and that the folds of the drape are supported on his arms in the bend of the elbows. This eliminates the risk of the drape falling below his waistline. (B) The completion of draping the Mayo stand.

infectants, page 57, the bactericidal action of the vapor of alcohol-formalin solution is beneficial in maintaining the sterility of the area above the level of the solution. (Fig. 44)

GUIDE TO THE HANDLING OF TRANSFER FORCEPS

Activity	*Principle*
When withdrawing the forceps from the germicide container, do not allow the forceps to touch the side or the top of the container.*	A sterile object becomes contaminated when it touches an unsterile area. (The area not covered with germicide solution cannot be considered to be sterile).
Keep the forceps' prongs or legs pointed downward at all times. If this is not done, germicide solution will flow toward the unsterile handle. Then when the forceps is returned to the correct position, the legs become contaminated.†	Gravity pulls the liquid downward.
When using the forceps, keep them within view at the level of the waist or above it.	A possibility of contamination exists when a sterile object is out of view.

* This problem is eliminated in the forceps illustrated in Figure 44 because of the inner coil and the movable inner metal collar.
† Even with the forceps illustrated in Figure 44 this is good practice, because with use it is possible for the lid to permit a leak of fluid.

Activity	*Principle*
Drop the sterile article gently on the sterile field; the forceps must not touch the field.	After an operation has begun, the sterile setup is sterile for that patient alone; should a sterile transfer forceps touch such a field, it is no longer sterile for any other field.
Do not use transfer forceps to pick up anything with an adhering base, such as petrolatum gauze. Should this occur, clean and resterilize the forceps.	An adhering substance on a forceps causes objects to cling to it.

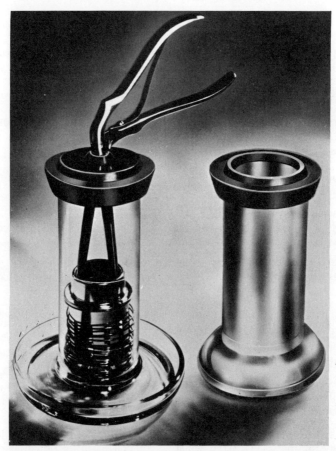

Fig. 43. Bard-Parker forceps. Clear container shows inside of container. Some surgeons prefer metal rather than transparent glass. Both are shown. (Becton, Dickinson and Company, Rutherford, N.J.)

Fig. 44. Bard-Parker transfer forceps. Forceps is being removed from container. Note that spring rises to top (see Fig. 43), which permits inner sterile cylinder to rise. This prevents the sterile forceps from touching the top outer guard. (Becton, Dickinson and Company)

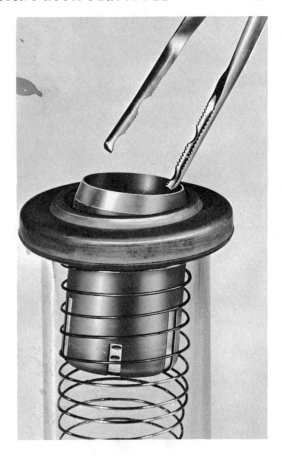

OPENING A STERILE PACKAGE

This may be done by placing the package on a table and undoing the wrapper in such a way that only the outside cover is touched by the circulating nurse. Or she may hold the package in her left hand and unwrap with the right hand.

The scrub nurse may take the offered package, or it may be dropped safely on a sterile field. The loose ends of the wrapper must be drawn back and away from the inner sterile package and the sterile field. The arm and the hands of the circulating nurse must not reach over the sterile field. (Fig. 45)

HANDLING A STERILE COVERED CONTAINER

The hazards of using sterile covered containers with multiple items must be understood. Each time the lid is removed there is a possibility of airborne contamination; hence, unnecessary or prolonged removal of the lid should be avoided. When several persons use a common container, the risk of contamination exists.

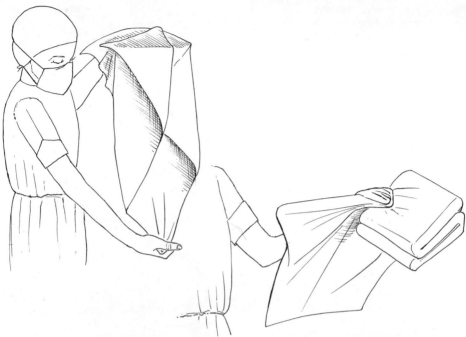

Fig. 45. (*Top*) The first step is unwrapping the package. (*Bottom*) The package completely unwrapped and ready to hand to a sterile nurse or to place on a sterile table.

To minimize these problems, each person using such a container must be thoroughly familiar with the handling of it. (Fig. 46)

GUIDE TO THE HANDLING OF A STERILE COVERED CONTAINER

Activity	*Principle*
Remove the lid only when necessary, and replace it as soon as possible.	The possibility of airborne contamination exists.
In removing the lid, hold it in such a way that the sterile undersurface faces downward.	Because of gravity, dust particles, etc., tend to fall downward.
If it is necessary to set the lid down, the sterile undersurface faces upward.	Contact with an unsterile surface contaminates a sterile object.
The rims of the lid and the container are considered as being unsterile.	Proximity to unsterile surfaces makes the rim of the lid and container a doubtful area. When sterility is questioned, consider the object (or field) as being contaminated.

Fig. 46. (*Above*) If the lid is held, it should be held with the inner surface downward to prevent contamination. (*Below*) If the lid is placed on a table, the outer surface is placed downward to prevent contamination to the inner surface. (Sutton, A. L.: Bedside Nursing Techniques, p. 90, Philadelphia, Saunders, 1964)

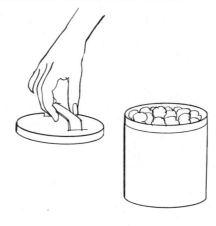

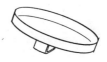

Activity	*Principle*
Unused sterile objects are not to be returned to the sterile container.	Air currents are capable of carrying contaminants.

Note: It is desirable to have all materials packaged in functional units.

POURING STERILE SOLUTIONS

Sterile flasks or bottles are covered with a top which fits over the outer edge of the container. To remove the cap, touch only the top outer surface and avoid touching the edge. If the flask or bottle has a pouring lip, such as the Pour-o-vac, sterile fluids can be dispensed safely.

When solutions are poured, the flask or pitcher must be held high enough so that the unsterile outside of the container or the hand of the pourer will not touch the receiving sterile basin. On the other hand, the flask should not be held so high that the solution will splash. When the flask is too warm to handle, special tongs are available to grasp the flask safely (Fig. 47).

REVIEW QUESTIONS:
1. What precautions should be taken to keep masks effective?
2. Which is more effective, the length of time one scrubs or the thoroughness with which one scrubs?
3. Evaluate the procedure for gowning and gloving in your hospital. Suggest areas of improvement.
4. Review the principles of draping as they apply to the draping of a Mayo stand.
5. What ways can the forceps described on page 102 be contaminated? Is there a weakness in the design of this forceps? Discuss.

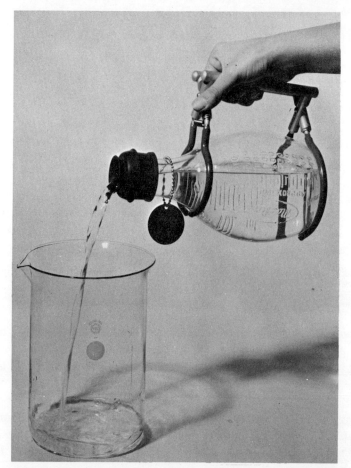

Fig. 47. By using special tongs hot solutions can be poured
safely. (The Macbick Company, Wilmington, Mass.)

Bibliography

Adams, R., and Fraser, R.: Plastic skin drapes, Am. J. Nurs. 59:845–847, June 1959.
Beck, W. C.: Justified faith in surgical drapes, Am. J. Surg. 105:560–562, April 1963.
Devlin, L.: One day in the life of a circulatory nurse in open heart work, A.O.R.N.J.
2:72–75, March–April 1964.
Prioleau, W. H.: Contamination resulting from incorrect drying of hands and careless
surgical attire, A.O.R.N.J. 2:62–66, September–October 1964.
———: Psychological difficulties in the maintenance of sterile technic, A.O.R.N.J.
1:61, November–December 1963.
Rockwell, V. T.: Surgical hand scrubbing, Am. J. Nurs. 63:75–81, June 1963.

UNIT **3**

The Surgical Patient

CHAPTER 7

PREPARATION OF THE ENVIRONMENT TO ENSURE PATIENT SAFETY

HOUSEKEEPING : LIGHTING : VENTILATION : TRAFFIC : ROOM
SETUP : SUCTION : CONDUCTIVITY

HOUSEKEEPING

Part of the orientation of employees to the operating room includes learning about the procedure book, its contents and use. Standard procedures are set up for all phases of cleaning and housekeeping as well as for surgical procedures.

Cleanliness and order are recognized as vitally important measures in the prevention of wound infection. Infection is bacterial-caused inflammation (see Infection, p. 41) and every precaution must be taken to eliminate as many bacteria in the environment as is possible.

The job of cleaning may be done by operating room porters or orderlies, nurse's aides, technicians, or by employees of the housekeeping staff who have been assigned to the operating room for this purpose. Direct supervision of the cleaning is done by the operating room nurse. She works directly with the auxiliary personnel, can instruct as well as observe, and by so doing can maintain the high standards of cleanliness necessary.

The standard procedure for disinfecting a room following a surgical case is followed conscientiously. Major cleaning of air ducts, vents, windows, storage closets and instrument cabinets is scheduled at regular time intervals, and strict adherence to this schedule is important. Specific routine procedures are completed after each case. Some are done daily; others, twice a week or weekly, according to the set standard procedure.

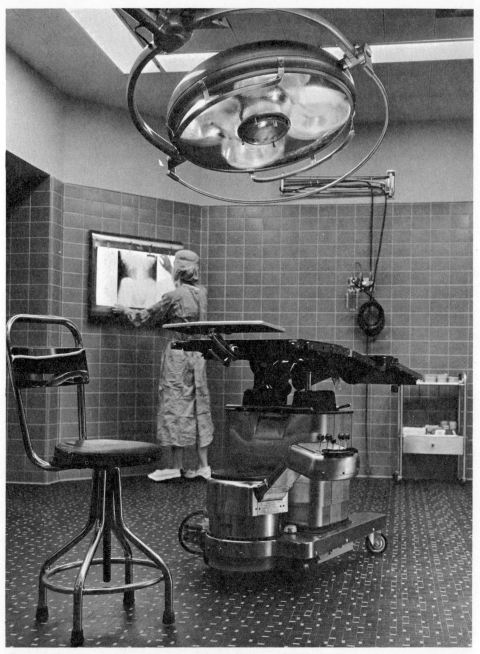

Fig. 48. Single overhead surgical light. Note the cove base as it approximates the wall for easy cleaning, the electrically controlled operating table (Castle T-5000), overhead boom conveying oxygen and nitrous oxide gases, x-ray transilluminator, wall suction, and conductive anesthetist's stool. On the right is an explosion-proof receptacle, conductive ceramic tile floor, conductive booties worn by the circulating nurse and the proper wearing of her headgear. (Wilmot Castle Company, Rochester, N.Y.)

After each case is completed, tables, stools, kick buckets, operating room pad and table are treated with a disinfectant wash. The operating room table is moved from its position in the center of the room so that the floor beneath it can be reached by the cleaning agent. Floors are mopped or flooded with the solution, and if flooded, then are vacuumed dry. The technic of dry dusting, sweeping or dust mopping spreads organisms from one surface to another by air currents and is an unsafe practice.

Each morning about a half hour before the surgery schedule begins in each operating room, the furniture is damp dusted with a disinfectant solution. Meticulous care and cleanliness can reduce the number of airborne infections. Although the environment cannot be sterilized, it can be kept at a level that is bacteriologically safe.

Suture ends may become twisted in the wheels of furniture and equipment and must be removed. Castors and wheels are lubricated at least once a month and more often if needed. Suction tubing and containers are removed to the clean-up area for cleaning and reprocessing and are replaced with fresh units.

The often forgotten places and equipment such as cabinet tops, tops of doors, stretchers and their wheels, table accessories, stirrup straps, bases and collars of kick buckets, ether screens, x-ray view boxes, etc., must be included in the clean-up process.

It is customary to have the "duties" of all personnel in the operating room procedure book. The duties of an orderly working from 7 A.M. to 3:30 P.M. may be quite different from those for an orderly working from 3:30 P.M. to 11 P.M. The procedure book should be used frequently by personnel to remind them of their many assigned duties until they are well oriented to their jobs. The co-ordinated efforts of all members of the nursing service team, each doing his job conscientiously, results in an immaculately clean surgery where each item is in its own place. The patient then is assured a safe surgical environment.

Care must be exercised in selecting the disinfectant used for cleaning purposes. It is mandatory that it not decrease the conductivity of floors, shoes and wheels of equipment, and it must be bacteriologically effective.

LIGHTING

The design of surgical lighting is essentially the specialized field of illuminating engineers and of surgeons. The surgeon has specific requirements for effectively illuminating the operative area. The type of light selected for use should conform to the requirements of the type of surgery to be performed. Other equipment in the operating room may limit the kind of light to be installed (observation galleries, TV, motion picture cameras, etc.).

The desirable features in the design of the light[1] are: ease of maneuverability, ability of the light to concentrate in a spot, the ability to travel horizontally and

1 Smith, Warwick: Planning the Surgical Suite, p. 142, New York, F. W. Dodge Corp., 1960.

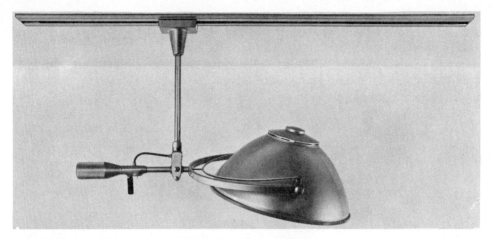

Fig. 49. The single-track overhead angle of the lamp is adjusted by the dependent black
handle. (AMSCO, American Sterilizer Company, Erie, Pa.)

vertically, ease of cleaning and maintenance, resistance to explosion, and low
temperature. The surgical light may be mounted on a track and secured in a recess
above the ceiling, with the track suspended in the operating room above the
operating room table, or there may be one or more lights on tracks to give lateral
illumination and adjustment for special types of surgery. Portable spotlights may
be used.

Whatever types of lights are selected, they must be firmly mounted so that there
is no danger of their falling on a patient, and they must be made of materials that
do not have crevices and uneven surfaces that could harbor bacteria.

The switch for the surgical light or lights usually is located adjacent to the
switches that control the general room lighting. General room lighting usually is
scattered over the ceiling in several places, giving adequate illumination for setting
up the room for surgery and for transferring the patient to the table. It is diffused
so that it does not shine in the patient's eyes, cause sharp glare from instruments or
linens, or produce dark corners in the room.

A special intensity-control switch (rheostat) is used with those lights that
provide high-intensity illumination. All surgical lights should be connected to the
emergency electrical supply, so that they would continue to function if a power
failure occurred.

Recently developed fiberoptics such as Satelight

provide a complementary source of illumination for deep-cavity surgical wounds or other
difficult-to-illuminate operative areas . . . utilizing a low-voltage light source to provide
a high-intensity light pattern.[2]

The Satelight consists of an optical fiber bundle made up of flexible, coated glass
fibers. The bundle has an over-all covering of steam-resistant plastic (see p. 71).

[2] AMSCO, American Sterilizer Company, Erie, Pa.

VENTILATION

The physical conditions within the operating room suite must be controlled if a suitable environment for surgery is to be provided. The most suitable control is the process of treating air so that temperature, humidity, cleanliness and distribution meet specific requirements.

Air conditioning is more expensive to install and maintain than any other kind of heating or ventilating system. Consequently, there still are hospitals that do not have it, or that have it in only limited areas of the surgical suite. Since no

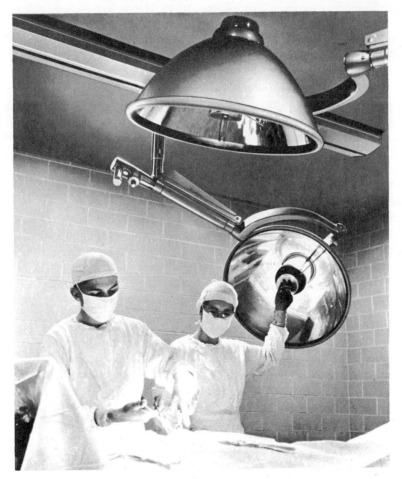

Fig. 50. Overhead lighting on dual tracks. Note that the nursing assistant can position the overhead light through the use of sterilized handles fastened to the light. Contact with the rim of the light must be avoided. (Wilmot Castle Company)

monetary evaluation of the advantages of air conditioning can be made, it is not possible to prove that it is necessary for the efficient operation of the suite. However, in some states air conditioning of a surgical suite is required by law, in some it is recommended by the Public Health Service, and it has been adopted by many public departments (for instance, Veterans Administration, Department of the Navy). Better hospitals provide air conditioning within their operating room suites.[3]

Fresh air intake ducts which supply the surgical suite should be placed so that air uncontaminated by hospital exhausts can be drawn into the system. The exhaust air from the surgical suite may contain pathogenic material and should be discharged in such a position that no hospital air intake will be contaminated from it. Air which is drawn into the fresh air intake contains a quantity of airborne particles, and it must be filtered before it is circulated through the system. It generally is agreed that some types of filters are more effective than others for the operating room suite.

Air conditioning is a highly technical process, and there is no need to describe it in detail. Suffice it to say that room temperature should be kept within a range of 68° to 80° F. The ideal is to equip each room with an individual control. Some thermostats may be remotely adjustable from a central control cabinet. There is general agreement that the figure of 55 per cent relative humidity (moisture) is satisfactory for the operating room suite. This figure is recommended to reduce the possibility of electrostatic discharge and, consequently, the likelihood of the explosion of combustible gases.

When the air distribution system provides slightly more air to each operating room than is exhausted from it, the rooms will be kept under positive pressure. This principle reduces the infiltration of odors and pathogenic materials from adjoining rooms and corridors.[4]

TRAFFIC

OPERATING ROOM PERSONNEL

Only authorized personnel are permitted in the restricted area of the operating room, and they must be garbed properly before they are allowed to enter. In the dressing rooms operating room personnel remove street clothes and place them in lockers. After showering they put on clean, freshly laundered scrub gowns or suits and conductive footwear, and then they are ready to enter the restricted area of the suite. A conductivity meter is used to check each person's electrical charge relative to the floor to ensure that he is safe to enter a "hazardous location" where a static spark could cause an explosion of anesthetic gases. Caps and masks usually

[3] Smith, Warwick: Planning the Surgical Suite, pp. 362–363, New York, F. W. Dodge Corp., 1960.
[4] Ibid., p. 373.

are put on from containers in the scrub-up area, or they may be located in the dressing room, in which case they are put on at the same time as the scrub garb.

When operations have been completed, surgeons return to the change area and prepare to leave the suite in their street clothes. Nurses and other nursing service personnel remain in the suite to prepare the rooms for the next cases. The traffic pattern for them includes the clean-up and disassembling area, etc.

Depending on the severity of the patient's condition, orderlies generally are assigned the task of transporting patients to and from the surgical suite and assisting in the transfer of patients from one conveyance to another. Often they help with the cleaning of the operating rooms between cases. Housekeeping personnel carry out the general cleaning of the suite.

VISITORS

Visitors are not permitted within the operating room unless there is specific reason for their presence. When they are present, their street clothes are exchanged for scrub garb, conductive coverings are placed over their shoes, and a cap and a mask are worn. A member of the surgical or nursing staff should accompany them and be responsible for them while they are in the suite. No visitor should be allowed to roam unattended because of the possibility of inadvertent contamination of a sterile field or supplies. In the event of a visiting surgeon or nurse, such exacting supervision may not be necessary, but they must comply with the existing policies, rules and regulations of the institution that they are visiting.

TV PERSONNEL

There is increasing use of closed-circuit TV for demonstration and teaching purposes. Yet many problems arise in its use. Cameras mounted on portable equipment and brought into the operating room must be operated there. This involves a thorough orientation of the TV technicians in aseptic technics used in the operating room. A break in technic could cause contamination of the field and thereby would pose a dangerous threat to the safety of the patient. A more acceptable plan is to have a camera hung from the ceiling of the operating room and controlled remotely from a station separated from the operating room, or a camera mounted outside the operating room and focused through a hole in the ceiling or the wall.

ENGINEERS

It is seldom necessary to have an engineer in a room to fix something that has broken or gone wrong while surgery is in progress. Usually, the services of the engineer can be scheduled when a surgery room is not being used. In either instance he must be properly attired in operating room garb just as are all persons who enter the restricted area. He is taught to avoid bringing in any more contamination within the surgery than is absolutely necessary. Cooperative relationships should be built between the two departments, and a schedule should be made up for routine preventive maintenance that is acceptable to both the operating room and the engineers. With such a plan in effect, there are few instances of an emergency nature which would require the services of an engineer when surgery was in progress.

In most hospitals it may be economically unsound for engineers to have special sets of tools to use only in the operating room. However, this is advisable, to prevent tools which have been contaminated elsewhere in the hospital from being brought into the operating room suite. When necessary, the tools must be cleaned as well as the areas where the engineer has been working. The engineer's typically greasy and grimy hands should be washed thoroughly before starting a repair job in the operating room.

X-RAY PERSONNEL

When the taking of x-ray pictures is planned as a part of an operation, the operating room supervisor schedules the request with the x-ray department. The x-ray technician assigned to the case appears in surgery properly attired (as are other personnel) at the appropriate time. If portable x-ray equipment must be moved into the suite, the machine (including the wheels) is thoroughly wiped down by the technician, using a detergent-germicide-soaked cloth. Protective lead aprons are worn by operating room personnel who must remain close to the patient while pictures are being taken. After the x-ray pictures have been taken, the plates are developed in either the operating room darkroom or the x-ray department.

The operating room supervisor usually conducts classes in aseptic practice for x-ray and laboratory personnel who are unfamiliar with these technics. Included in the classes are instructions for wearing masks, caps and scrub garb and for working in an aseptic environment.

LABORATORY PERSONNEL

Personnel from the laboratory have occasion to come to the operating room for technical consultation (for example, the nature of tissue) or to take specimens such as blood and other materials for immediate analysis. A minimum of equipment is brought into the surgery room. Trays or boxes of supplies are left on a table in the corridor.

ROOM SETUP

PHYSICAL PLAN OF THE OPERATING ROOM

Today it is generally considered to be economically sound to have all operating rooms equipped similarly and of a size that permits them to be used for major or minor surgery. Specialty equipment such as eye, "neuro," plastic, etc., could be stocked on wheeled carts and brought into any room when needed. In a modern operating room there should be no less than 20 x 20 feet of clear space,[5] not including the built-in cabinets across one wall. (Figs. 51, 52)

Furniture placement may vary somewhat from one institution to another. If storage-room space for large equipment is not available, units such as an electro-diathermy machine may be kept in a corner of the operating room. This practice is questionable, however, because another piece of equipment is present to gather dust and to be kept clean.

Cystoscopic Room. This is equipped with a special table for urologic procedures, built-in x-ray facilities and special irrigating apparatus. Space is provided for the storing of scopes (either in their boxes or ready for use after gas sterilization) and all the accessories and equipment needed for urologic work. Since urologic patients do not have a surgical incision, this room is not a part of the operating room proper. It is located preferably near the entrance of the operating room suite and may open out into the unrestricted part of the operating room corridor. *Major urologic surgery* is done in a major surgery room.

Cast Room. The routine application of plaster casts should be done in a cast room located elsewhere in the hospital, usually somewhere near the emergency room and the x-ray department. Plaster dust should be excluded entirely from the operating room suite if possible, although some casts are applied in the operating room as a part of orthopedic surgery when immobilization is desired. It sometimes becomes necessary to have a cast room in the operating room suite, but it should not be used for outpatients, for the changing of inpatient's casts, or for the reduction of simple fractures not requiring anesthesia or surgery. This room usually is located adjacent to the particular operating room that is equipped to handle orthopedic patients. However, by using a mobile, well-equipped plaster cart, casts can be applied in any room.

Special Operating Rooms. These can be designed to accommodate cardiac surgery. The amount of equipment used and the number of technicians required make it difficult to perform extensive cardiac surgery in a standard-sized room.

PERSONNEL ACTIVITIES IN THE OPERATING ROOM SETUP

When the scrub assistant has scrubbed and goes into the operating room to prepare the sterile tables for the case, sterile gown and gloves are donned from individual open packages placed either on the "prep" table (before the tray has been opened) or on the foot of the operating table. The wrappers then are discarded in the linen hamper by the circulating nurse.

The circulating nurse moves the furniture to be draped away from the wall, opens the packs, assists with supplying sutures and other needed items to the

[5] Gifford, D. L.: Basic planning of the O.R. suite, Hosp. Progr. 44: May 1963.

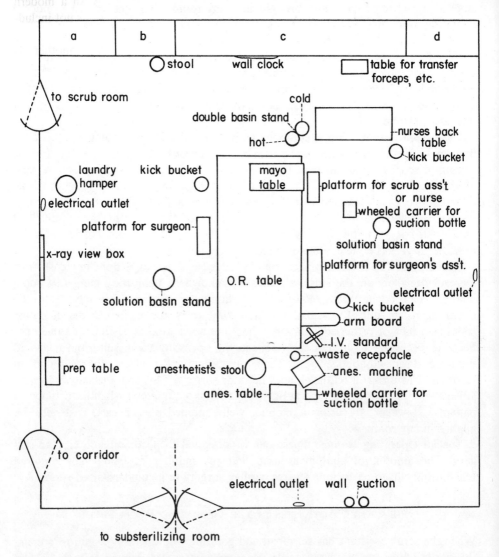

Fig. 51. A major surgery room set up with the furniture in place for a general surgery procedure. (*Top*, a) Unsterile supply closet; (b) desk with overhead cabinets; (c) sterile supply cabinets; (d) table accessories storage cabinet.

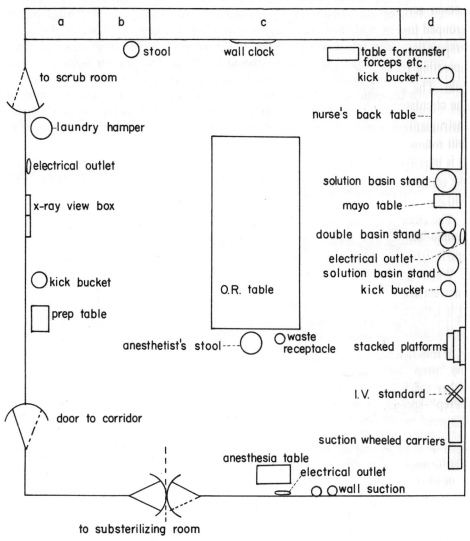

Fig. 52. The same room as that in Figure 51 after the room has been cleaned, and the
furniture has been restored to out-of-the-way positions. (*Top,* a) Unsterile
supply closet; (b) desk with overhead cabinets; (c) sterile supply cabinets;
(d) table accessories storage cabinet.

person scrubbed, and counts sponges with her. The furniture to be draped is grouped together in one place in the room so that traffic in and out of the doors or preparations by the anesthesia department and the placing of the patient on the operating room table do not in any way jeopardize the preparation of the sterile field. The sterile tables are near the sterile supply closets (Fig. 51a) to assist the circulator in helping the scrub assistant to set up. The positioning of the sterile instruments, linens, sponges, specimen basin and other needed supplies on the table will follow the routine procedure used in the institution in which one is employed. It is important that standard table setups be used so that if another person becomes the scrub assistant, she knows where everything is placed and can continue assisting without confusion or delay.

The circulator pours sterile water from a sterile flask into one of the basins in the double-basin stand. This gives the scrub assistant a place to rinse off suture tubes and instruments that may have been in a chemical disinfectant.

When nonexplosive anesthetic gas mixtures are used, the patient may be anesthetized in an induction room and then transferred into the operating room. It is important that suction and oxygen be available in the induction room as well as the operating room.

When the anesthetist indicates that the patient is ready for further preparation, the "prep" table is moved into a position convenient to the operative site, and either the interne or the circulating nurse prepares the skin (Chap. 8, p. 159). "Prep" sponges are discarded in a plastic liner in a kick bucket and then are removed and returned to the used "prep" tray. After skin preparation the patient is draped (Chap. 8, p. 163), and the furniture is moved into position for use. Platforms (low, wide-based, metal footstools with conductive tips) are distributed if needed, kick buckets are rolled into positions where they are easily reached by the team members, and the solution basin stands are moved to a convenient distance for use and yet far enough from the backs of the team members to prevent contamination. The Mayo table is placed over the patient in a position comfortable for the surgeon and the nurse without pressure on any part of the patient's body. The adjustment of the table is done from underneath the Mayo table drapes by the circulator while the scrub assistant guides it from above into the proper position.

The circulating nurse helps with moving the furniture into place but touches only unsterile surfaces, while the scrub assistant handles only the sterile surfaces. When these preparations are complete, the surgeon and his assistant are ready to make the incision.

SUCTION

Suction is needed by the surgeon to remove fluids from the wound and by the anesthetist to remove secretions from the patient's throat so that a clear airway during the induction and the administration of anesthesia can be maintained. This requires two suction units in each operating room. The most acceptable means of providing this is a central piped system in which the suction comes from a wall installation equipped with a regulator, a gauge and a bottle that is supported at the wall adjacent to the installation. To this bottle is attached, by means of flexible tubing, a bottle set on a wheeled carrier located near the operating room table. The second suction unit, that used by the anesthetist, likewise is connected to the central system. The bottle for this apparatus is placed near the anesthesia table so that secretions drawn into it can be observed by the anesthetist. (Fig. 53)

The scrub assistant attaches the sterile tubing to the sterile drape over the patient so that the suction tip is available to the surgeon. The other end of the tubing is handed to the circulating nurse, who attaches it to the inlet side of the suction bottle on the wheeled carrier.

In some instances an attempt has been made to connect both the surgeon's and the anesthetist's suction to one bottle by using a Y-type connector to the bottle on the wheeled carrier. This is not satisfactory, because if both needed maximum suction at the same time, neither would have enough. Therefore, separate units should be provided.

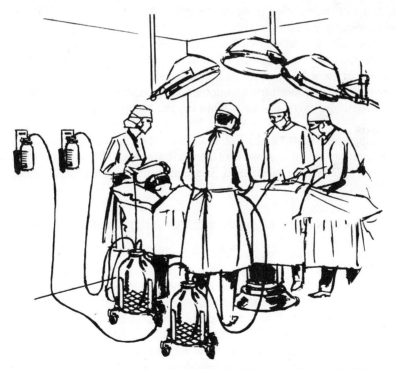

Fig. 53. Two suction units, as described in the text. (National Cylinder Gas Division of Chemetron Corporation, Conshohocken, Pa.)

CONDUCTIVITY

PRINCIPLES OF COMBUSTION

Combustion (burning or explosion) is a chemical change that occurs with sufficient rapidity to produce heat and light. It requires (1) a combustible substance, (2) a supporter of combustion, and (3) a source of ignition.

A *combustible substance* is anything which is capable of burning. The *supporter of combustion* is oxygen. In the administration of anesthesia, oxygen is supplied in varying concentrations from

---

FLAMMABLE ANESTHETIC AGENTS

Cyclopropane

Divinyl ether (Vinethene)

Ethyl ether

Ethyl chloride

Ethylene

---

pure (100%) to less concentrated amounts diluted in air. Oxygen is found also in chemical combination with nitrogen in the gas, nitrous oxide.

An *ignition source*—that is, something to start the reaction—in the operating room may be found in fixed and portable electrical equipment, open flames, heated objects, and an accumulation of static electricity. These must be carefully controlled to avoid fires and explosions.

Static electricity is that form of electricity which can be seen and heard when the fur of a cat is stroked. Sparks of static electricity can be seen and heard also if one stands in front of a mirror in a dark room and brushes the hair vigorously. Most people have at some time or another slid across a car seat to get out of the car and in so doing have placed a hand on the metal door and received a slight shock.

In the operating room a small spark from static electricity could serve as a source of ignition for an explosion of flammable gases. The buildup of an electrostatic charge is prevented when there is a conductive pathway that drains it off as it is generated.

MEASURES TO ELIMINATE THE POSSIBILITY OF COMBUSTION

Equipment and Floor. A good conductive floor prevents the accumulation of electrostatic charges by providing a path of conductivity between all persons and equipment making contact with it. Electrically conductive floors, needed to prevent explosions in the operating suite and in all areas where anesthesia is administered, are designed by engineers who are aware of the explosive hazards involved. Manufacturers, architects and builders concerned with hospital design supply materials and construction which conform with the modern safety code requirements.[6] The resistance of the conductive floor is tested at specified intervals to insure safety.

[6] Safe Practice for Hospital Operating Rooms, Bulletin No. 56, National Fire Protection Association, 1962.

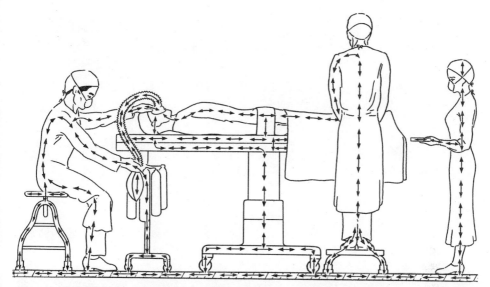

Fig. 54. The conductive pathway that permits equalization of electrostatic charges is illustrated by the double-headed arrows. The conductive floor is the common pathway. Conductive casters, conductive rubber feet and conductive footwear establish electrical connection with the high-resistance floor. The patient is connected by means of the anesthesia machine and the conductive strap fixed to the metal table. Thus, all objects and persons are electrically interconnected. Differences of potential are equalized before hazardous accumulation occurs. (Walter, C. W.: Anesthetic explosions: a continuing threat, Anesthesiology 25:510, 1964, and adapted from Hudenburg, R.: New recommendations for the control of operating room explosion hazards, Hospitals, December 1949)

(It must be more than 25,000 ohms as measured between two electrodes placed 3 feet apart anywhere on the floor.)[7]

Safe furniture is made of metal or other electrically conductive materials, and electrical contact with the floor is established through conductive leg tips (on stools or platforms), casters (on tables, basin stands, electrical equipment, etc.) and wheels (on stretchers).

A good conductive floor is worthless from a safety point of view if the equipment used does not make proper electrical contact with it. Equipment properly equipped with electrically conductive contact with the floor can create hazards if the point of contact (the wheels, the casters or the leg tips) is insulated with dirt, dust, wax, soap, bits of broken glass from suture tubes or ampules, ends of sutures, or layers of blood or other body secretions. The contact point must be kept clean and free

[7] Thomas, G. J.: Fire and explosion hazards with flammable anesthetics and their control, J. Nat. Med. Assoc. 52, No. 6:401, November 1960.

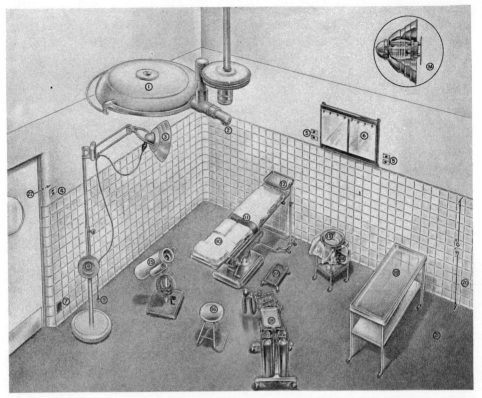

Fig. 55. View of an operating room illustrating coordination of structure and equipment to decrease the hazard of sparks due to power and electrostatic causes.

(1) Ceiling-suspended surgical light is wired in conventional manner and may be
fitted with (2) ordinary switch suitable for nonhazardous location.

(3) Explosion-proof spotlight. The lamp is enclosed in a strong housing ventilated
through porous radiator (3A). The metal frame is grounded. The casters are conductive
to provide leakage path for electrostatic charge generated while moving the light when
it is disconnected.

(4) Wall switch for ceiling-mounted surgical light. Enclosed single-pole switch and
conventional wiring for nonhazardous location above the 5-foot level.

(5) Receptacles for anesthetizing location plug supplied through isolation trans-
formers need not be explosion-proof if located above the 5-foot level.

(6) View box above 5-foot level connected to ungrounded distribution system.
Ordinary switch is permissible.

(7) Explosion-proof receptacle for anesthetizing location plug.

(8) Reel to prevent kinking of cord.

(9) Anesthetizing location plug interchangeably used in either 5 or 7.

(10) Operating table has unpainted metal top and conductive casters. Sponge rubber mattress is enclosed in conductive cover.

(11) Conductive strap connected to metal frame of table bridges bedding that may
insulate patient.

(12) All metal instrument stand has conductive casters.

Fig. 55 (Continued)

(13) Metal basin is connected to conductive system through (14) moistened drape. Solution is initially poured over rim of basin to moisten drape.

(15) Explosion-proof electrocardioscope.

(16) Unpainted metal stool.

(17) Footstool with conductive top and feet.

(18) Anesthesia machine is fitted with a conductive rubber gas transmission system and conductive casters.

(19) The metal instrument table is conductive when tested by placing an electrode on its top and another on the conductive floor.

(20) Dado to 5-foot level demarks extent of anesthetizing location.

(21) Conductive floor with resistance high enough to mitigate the shock hazard.

(22) Switches for conventionally grounded circuits are located outside the anesthetizing location. (Walter, C. W.: Anesthetic explosions: a continuing threat, Anesthesiology 25:512, 1964, and adapted from Hudenburg, R.: New recommendations for the control of operating room explosion hazards, Hospitals, December 1949)

of such debris. Otherwise static electricity can accumulate on that particular piece of equipment.

Since flammable gases tend to remain near the floor, electrical receptacles less than 5 feet above the floor should be explosion-proof.

All electrical equipment used in the operating room should be examined by the engineering department and not released until such equipment is declared to be safe from electrical or mechanical spark hazard.

Only *cotton* blankets should be used in the operating room. These blankets should not be warmed, because warming removes moisture, and moisture discourages the formation of static charges. Wool, silk or synthetic materials, such as rayon, orlon and nylon, or cotton *with* nylon or dacron, should be prohibited in anesthetizing locations because of their static potential. If a slight leak of combustible gas were to occur, a static discharge resulting from removal of the cover could ignite it.

Operating room table pads and pillows are covered with conductive rubber sheeting, and cotton covers and sheets are used. The cotton sheet acts as an insulator from the conductive pad cover but is universally accepted for esthetic reasons and for the sake of cleanliness. Walter[8] recommends that a conductive strap fixed permanently to the metal frame of the table, where it can be placed across the bare skin of the patient's shoulders or leg to bridge the insulating textile, be used for safety.

Oils, waxes, detergents, etc., which, when applied to the floor, reduce its conductivity, should be prohibited.

Personnel. Perhaps the one most important point in eliminating explosive hazards is the education of operating room personnel. To begin with, each person who works in the operating room wears the prescribed clothing and conductive shoes or boots (see p. 87). Shoes are tested on the conductometer before the restricted area

[8] Walter, C. W.: Electrostatics in the operating room, Hospital Topics, September 1953.

is entered. The soles (as well as the tops) are cleaned daily to keep them safe.

Smoking is restricted to dressing rooms and lounges, where the doors leading to the corridor are closed.

Moving a patient from one area to another while a flammable anesthetic is being administered is prohibited.

Since the most hazardous explosion location extends from a radius of 2 feet from the anesthesia machine and the patient's head and a similar distance above the floor,[9] personnel must be taught to stay away from the patient's head and the anesthetist's machines. The traffic pattern within the operating room should be at the sides and the foot of the operating room table and not directly behind the anesthetist.

Environment. It is commonly agreed that an atmosphere of high humidity prevents the accumulation of static electricity and thereby eliminates the explosions that could occur. In fact, most authoritative sources recommend a humidity of at least 55 per cent in the operating room. In those suites which have air conditioning and humidity controls, this is the humidity usually observed.

Open flames from Bunsen burners, alcohol lamps, cautery, cigarettes or pipes can serve as a source of ignition. Flammable antiseptics such as alcohol, acetone, ether, etc., should not be applied to the patient's skin when a flammable gas or a diathermy unit is in operation. Special precautions are taken when a cautery or electrical diathermy is used.

REVIEW QUESTIONS:

1. Discuss the relationship between housekeeping practices and wound infection.
2. Describe the desirable features in the design of surgery lights and explain why these features aid illumination of the surgical field.
3. At what temperature and per cent of humidity is the operating room kept?
4. Describe the basic operating room traffic pattern in your hospital.
5. What is your responsibility in relation to visitors in the operating room?
6. Why is suction needed by both the surgeon and the anesthetist during surgery?
7. List the preventive measures taken to reduce explosive hazards.
8. What rules of conduct do all personnel follow to help to decrease explosive hazards?

Bibliography

Barrett, R. H.: Explosion hazards in the operating room, Hospital Topics 33:86–88, October 1955.
Creber, I.: Safety measures in the operating room, Nurs. Outlook 6:528–531, September 1958.
Flammable Anesthetics, Code 1962, NFPA No. 56, Boston, National Fire Protection Assoc., 1964.
Gifford, D. L.: Basic planning of the O.R. suite, Hosp. Progr. 44: May, 1963.

[9] Walter, C. W.: Anesthetic explosions: a continuing threat, Anesthesiology 25:505–514, 1964.

Safe Practice for Hospital Operating Rooms, Bulletin No. 56, Boston, National Fire
    Protection Assoc., 1962.
Smith, Warwick: Planning the Surgical Suite, New York, F. W. Dodge Corp., 1960.
Thomas, G. J.: Fire and explosion hazards with flammable anesthetics and their control,
    J. Nat. Med. Assoc. 52, No. 6:597–403, November 1960.
Walter, C. W.: Electrostatics in the operating room, Hospital Topics, September 1953.
_____: Anesthetic explosions: a continuing threat, Anesthesiology 25:505–514, 1964.

THE PATIENT
APPROACHING SURGERY

SURGERY BASED ON NEED : PRELIMINARY PHYSICAL AND
MENTAL PREPARATION : IMMEDIATE PREOPERATIVE PREPARA-
TION : PREANESTHETIC MEDICATION : TRANSPORTATION OF THE
PATIENT TO THE OPERATING ROOM : RECEPTION OF THE
PATIENT IN THE OPERATING ROOM : ANESTHESIA : ANESTHETIC
AIDS : THE OPERATING TABLE : POSITIONING THE PATIENT :
PREPARATION OF THE OPERATIVE AREA : PATIENT DRAPING

SURGERY BASED ON NEED

When it is decided that a person needs to have an operation, his immediate reaction
usually is to ask: "Is surgery necessary? When should it be done? How long will
it be before I can resume a fairly normal life?" and many other questions.

CATEGORIES

For explanatory purposes, the surgeon often classifies or categorizes surgery as
follows:[1]

1. *Emergency*. These conditions require immediate attention, and the individual
should be taken to the hospital without delay. Some examples are:

[1] Adapted from Rothenberg, R. E.: Understanding Surgery, pp. 6–7, New York, Pocket Books,
Inc., 1955.

Extensive burns	Strangulated hernia
Major bone fractures	Urinary bladder obstruction
Fractured skull	Severe bleeding from any cavity
Gunshot wounds	Serious eye injuries
Stab wounds	Acute intestinal obstruction

2. *Urgent.* These conditions require prompt attention, and the individual should plan for hospital admission within 24 to 48 hours. Some examples are:

Cancer	Kidney or ureteral stones
Acute infection of gallbladder	Bleeding hemorrhoids
Bleeding uterine tumors	

3. *Required.* These conditions require an operation but do not demand immediate or prompt treatment. The individual should plan for hospital admission within a few weeks or months. Some examples are:

Tonsil removal	Gallbladder inflammation without
Cataracts of the eye	acute infection
Prostate conditions without bladder	Thyroid operations
obstruction	Bone deformities
Spinal fusion	Tumors of the uterus

4. *Elective.* These are conditions which should be operated upon, but in all probability the failure to have the surgery performed will not result in a catastrophe. Some examples are:

Cleft palate and harelip	Vaginal repair procedures
operations	Simple hernia
Repair of burn scars	Superficial cysts

5. *Optional.* These conditions would benefit by surgery, but surgery is not essential. An example is plastic surgery (cosmetic).

PRELIMINARY PHYSICAL AND MENTAL PREPARATION

ADMISSION

Preoperative preparation of a patient often is begun before the person enters the hospital. His physician describes in general what he will experience. Throughout his hospital stay he will be given the opportunity to ask questions that concern him. The nurse, the social worker, the physician, the nutritionist and the clergyman are available to assist and to direct him. If his problems should require the aid of other specialists, arrangements will be made for their help.

In addition to the admission requirements, it is desirable to obtain the address and the telephone number of his nearest relative or friend. This is kept in a convenient place on his chart. Usually, some form of identification, such as a wristband, is fastened to the patient for the duration of his hospital stay. On it are his complete name, the name of the physician and perhaps the service, the room number and the hospital number. (This later serves as one form of identification of the proper patient at the time he is admitted to the operating room.) He then is assigned to his bed, the choice of which should be made with his condition and preferences in mind. Psychologically, it is better for him to be placed near someone who is cheerful and recovering from surgery than near one who has dissimilar interest or is pessimistic or quite ill.

After admission the patient is given a physical examination by his physician, and further plans for his preoperative care are initiated. These may include diagnostic studies and supportive therapy, such as attention to his fluid and nutritional needs. His temperature, pulse, respiration, blood pressure and weight are recorded.

OPERATIVE PERMIT

A written consent permitting the administration of anesthesia and the surgeon to operate is a necessary legal procedure. Before the patient signs this permit, he has a right to know the nature of the operation and what to expect after it. It is the surgeon's responsibility to explain this to the patient. If the patient is of legal age and in full control of his mental faculties, he may sign his own permit. If he is a minor, not responsible or unconscious, his nearest adult relative assumes this responsibility. A patient may place an X on the permit if he is not able to write, provided that two adults sign as witnesses.

PREOPERATIVE CARE

Any individual who is to come to the operating room for surgery is required to have special preparation. This is done so that he will have his operation with the least amount of risk, discomfort and fear and will recover from it with a minimum of pain and other complications. He also should have an understanding of how he can assist in speeding his recovery and convalescence. Variously included in preoperative care are:

1. A complete *bath* and *shaving* of the skin (described on pp. 134, 135) in a generous area around the operative site.

2. An *enema.* This treatment often is ordered to evacuate the contents of the gastrointestinal tract, which would cause nausea and vomiting during induction and emergence from anesthesia and also might produce undue strain at the incision site postoperatively during vomiting, distention or defecation.

3. *Fasting.* By withholding food and fluids for several hours before the operation, the patient accepts the anesthetic agent more easily, and the surgeon is able to perform better surgery.

4. *Sedatives and narcotics.* Because of natural anxieties and to ensure a good night's sleep, a barbiturate (sleeping pill) generally is prescribed the night before surgery. Then about 1 or 2 hours before the operation a narcotic such as morphine or Demerol is given to relax and to dull the patient's sensations. At the same time a medication such as atropine or scopolamine also is given to minimize or to reduce secretions.

5. *Insertion of a nasogastric tube.* In certain types of abdominal operations,

particularly those on the intestinal tract, it is necessary to have a long rubber or plastic tube inserted through the nose into the esophagus and the stomach. The tube is fastened in place and aids in removing fluid and gas which can be uncomfortable.

6. *Administration of intravenous fluids, plasma and blood transfusions.* Often it is necessary to provide the nutritional, blood and electrolyte (special chemicals) needs of the patient by means of an intravenous infusion or a blood transfusion. In many instances the condition which is to be corrected by surgery has caused an imbalance or a deficiency of these elements. Such a condition and the preoperative fasting of the patient might supply factors that would contribute to postoperative complications. The administration of fluids and blood directly into the vein may be started any time before surgery and may continue to be supplied during and after the operation.

7. *Instruction in postoperative exercise.* Depending on the operation, it may be helpful to teach the patient before the operation how to perform certain exercises and maneuvers which he will be expected to perform postoperatively. These may include coughing, turning, deep breathing, practice in using special equipment, etc.

8. *Psychological and socioeconomic assistance.* The fears or worries of a patient may seriously affect his anesthetic induction and actual recovery from surgery. Therefore, opportunity is given to patients to receive help with such problems. If the problem concerns adequate care for his family while he is hospitalized, or if he has financial and job difficulties related to his illness, the medical social worker may give him guidance. If his fears relate to his condition and subsequent surgery, these may be explored by the nurse, surgeon, anesthesiologist, nutritionist, psychologist and clergyman.

A common practice is for the anesthesiologist to visit the patient the night before surgery to discuss the nature of the anesthetic to be administered, check the condition of his heart and lungs, answer any questions and allay any fears pertaining to anesthesia. In some hospitals an operating room nurse or nursing student also visits the patient and reviews the events of the operative day as they concern the patient in an effort to dispel some of the fears of the unknown, to give him an opportunity to ask questions, and, later, to enable him to know a familiar face in the operating room on the day of his surgery.

SKIN PREPARATION

The purpose of skin preparation preoperatively is to render the skin as clean and free of bacteria as possible without causing irritation or damage to the skin, without impairing its natural protective function, and without interfering with subsequent wound healing.[2]

The nature of skin has been discussed on page 89. Since the surgeon gains access to the source of the patient's difficulty through the skin, it becomes apparent that optimum cleanliness of the skin is paramount if infection is to be avoided. Because it is impossible to sterilize skin, the careful removal of hair and the con-

[2] Knocke, F. J., and Knocke, L. S.: Orthopaedic Nursing, p. 279, Philadelphia, Davis, 1951.

scientious use of prescribed soaps and antiseptics are advocated to render the skin as clean as possible.

For patients who are able to aid in their own preparation well in advance of surgery, it is recommended that they bathe with an antiseptic soap. Here the limitations of antibacterial soap must be recognized. For example, soap with hexachlorophene needs to be used for several days, since its action is slow and cumulative; furthermore, the use of regular soap or an alcohol solution or lotion on the skin inactivates the hexachlorophene. Another example of a limitation is that of quaternary ammonium compounds; when used on the skin as a bactericidal agent, they completely lose their effectiveness in the presence of soap.

A highly effective skin antiseptic that can be used for skin "prepping" is an iodine compound, polyvinylpyrrolidone-iodine complex, or PVP-I.* This antibacterial agent has been shown to destroy bacteria, viruses, fungi, protozoa and yeasts, is low in toxicity and has prolonged action.

Skin Shaving. A liberal area including and surrounding the operative site is shaved of hair to aid in reducing sources of contamination. Figure 56 illustrates the extent of the area to be prepared for some of the more common operations. Skin shaving may be done by a special "prep" team, by personnel on the patient's unit, or by a member of the operating room team. When there is a question concerning the site of operation, it is advisable to consult the surgeon. Skin shaving may be done the evening before surgery or preferably in the designated preparation room immediately prior to the operation. Hair removed from the head is cut first before the final shaving is done; the cut hair is collected in a bag, labeled with the patient's name and saved (for possible later use, such as the making of a wig or for religious requirements, etc.).

The patient is told about the shaving procedure, placed in a convenient comfortable position and not exposed unduly. Soap solution should be applied at a comfortable temperature. Proper lighting and skill with a sharp razor will aid in producing a clean hairless area. Commercially made disposable "prep" trays are available which contain nonabsorbent and absorbent towels, cotton balls or gauze sponges, lathering sponge with hexachlorophene or measured amounts of antiseptic soap, and disposable razors. Such trays, available from several suppliers, ensure that each patient has individualized equipment.

Depilatory Cream. Chemical compounds (creams) to remove hair have been perfected sufficiently to make them safe for preparing the skin of the surgical patient. Long hairs may be cut before applying the cream as an economy measure, since less cream would be required; however, cutting hairs in the operating room area must be done very cautiously to eliminate loose flying hair, which would be a source of contamination.

The depilatory cream usually comes in a collapsible metal tube and is expressed on the body surface. The cream is spread to a smooth layer of about ¼" in depth over the entire operative site by a wooden tongue blade or a gloved hand. After the

* Povidone-iodine, N.N.D. 1964.

cream has been allowed to remain on the skin for 10 minutes, it is scraped off gently with the tongue blade or multiple moistened gauze sponges. When all cream and hair have been removed, the skin then is washed with soap and water and patted dry.

There are several advantages to using a depilatory cream for preoperative skin preparation. A clean, smooth and intact skin is produced. Scrapes, abrasions, cuts and poor hair removal are eliminated. It is more comfortable for the patient, since he is less apprehensive and often finds this method relaxing. There is even the possibility of the patient preparing himself in selected operative procedures. Depilatory creams are more effective and safer for use on uncooperative or agitated patients. This method is no more expensive than other methods. A disadvantage is that a few patients have had some transient skin reactions involving rectal and scrotal areas.

Preparation of Operative Field (Fig. 56). *Cranial Operations.* Obtain specific instructions from the surgeon as to the extent of shaving that is necessary.

Thyroid and Neck Operations. Shave the anterior neck from under the chin to the nipple line. The whole area should be shaved back to the hair line and to meet the bed line when the patient is lying in the supine position.

Breast Amputation (mastectomy). Shave the axilla on the affected side. Skin preparation should extend from above the clavicle to the umbilicus, from beyond the midline anteriorly to beyond the midline posteriorly. Particular care should be taken in cleansing the folds underneath the breast.

Operations on the Abdomen. Shave from the nipple line in males and from below the breast in females to and including the pubic area. Laterally, shaving should extend to the anterior axillary line. Particular care should be taken in cleansing the umbilicus and the inguinal creases.

Inguinal Hernia. Shave the lower abdomen from the umbilicus downward, including the suprapubic area and about 6 inches of the upper thigh on the affected side. Particular attention should be paid to cleansing the groin.

Operations on the Lower Bowel and the Rectum. Shave the entire abdomen, as for any abdominal operation, and in addition prepare the perineum as for any anal operation.

Anal Operations. Shave the area for a distance of about 10 inches from the anus. A suprapubic preparation is not necessary in male patients, but a partial perineal shave should be carried out in female patients.

Amputations. The area should be shaved and the skin cleansed for a distance of about 12 inches above and below the proposed site of amputation. It is necessary for the nurse to know where the amputation is to be performed. Thus, in gangrene of the foot the amputation often is through the thigh, and therefore it is necessary to prepare the thigh.

Skin Grafts. Shave both anterior thighs or the area from which a graft is to be taken. Request instructions.

Operations on the Spine. Shave and prepare the skin for an area of 12 inches above and below the site of operation. Ask the surgeon for instructions.

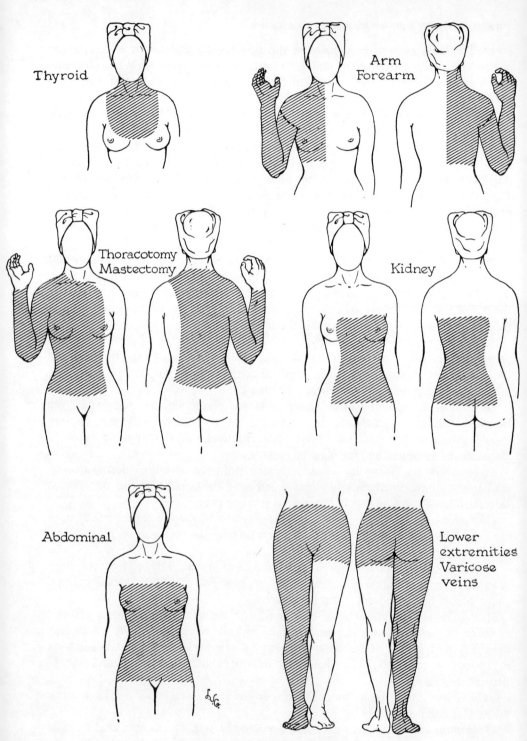

Thyroid

Arm
Forearm

Thoracotomy
Mastectomy

Kidney

Abdominal

Lower
extremities
Varicose
veins

Fig. 56. (*Caption on facing page*)

IMMEDIATE PREOPERATIVE PREPARATION

The patient is summoned to the operating room about 20 to 30 minutes before the anesthesia is to be started. In this interval he is asked to wear the hospital gown, and in some hospitals he may be required to wear long leggings. The hair is covered with a cap. All hairpins and bobbypins will have been removed from the hair of women. If the hair is long, it is plaited in two braids. The patient voids to empty the bladder and prevent incontinence later, and the amount and the time are recorded on the Preoperative Checklist (Fig. 57). The mouth is inspected for loose objects such as gum or candy; dentures or loose bridges also are removed to prevent respiratory obstruction during induction of anesthesia. Jewelry may not be worn to the operating room; however, a ring which cannot be removed is tied with gauze bandage and fastened around the wrist (Fig. 58). Any articles of value—dentures, jewelry, prostheses such as artificial eyes or legs, money, etc.—are placed in an envelope and given to the head nurse for safekeeping. Colored nail polish usually is removed from two fingers so that the anesthetist will be able to detect early signs of circulatory impairment.

PREANESTHETIC MEDICATION

Special medications are given the patient at this time, usually hypodermically, to assist him in accepting the anesthesia more smoothly. These drugs can be grouped in three categories: (1) the opiates, such as morphine, and synthetic narcotics, such as Metopon, methadone, and meperidine (Demerol); (2) barbiturates, such as pentobarbital (Nembutal) and secobarbital (Seconal Sodium); (3) belladonna derivatives—atropine and scopolamine; and (4) tranquilizers, such as chlorpromazine (Thorazine) and antihistaminics, such as promethazine hydrochloride (Phenergan).

The drugs in the first two groups tend to relax and allay apprehension, thus raising the pain threshold (tolerance for pain); fear lowers the pain threshold. Relaxation lowers the body metabolism, and therefore not so much anesthetic agent is needed. Those in the third group, belladonna derivatives, reduce the amount of secretions in the mouth and the respiratory tract. They also minimize spasm such as laryngospasm, thereby maintaining the clear airway so necessary for normal breathing. Those in the last group are used to relieve apprehension, to reduce the possibility of vomiting and to supply the effects of a sedative.

The choice of drugs is determined on an individual basis. This is affected by the patient's condition, age, weight and the anesthetic to be used. Preanesthetic medications are given exactly when ordered, so that they are having their maximum effect during anesthesia induction.

Fig. 56. Diagrams indicating the fields of preparation for common aseptic operations. (Harkins, H. N., et al.: Surgery, Principles and Practice, ed. 2, p. 218, Philadelphia, Lippincott, 1961, and there redrawn from similar diagrams in Moseley's Textbook of Surgery, ed. 2, St. Louis, Mosby, 1955)

Patient: _____ Ward _____

	Remarks:	YES	NO
1. Operative area prepared			
2. Operative area inspected by head nurse or supervisor			
3. Jewelry a. Removed			
b. Tied on			
4. False teeth removed			
5. Hair prepared — covered if necessary Hairpins removed			
6. Voided or catheterized Amount:			
Time:			
7. Preanesthetic medication Time:			
8. Side rails applied after giving preanesthetic medication			
9. Pulse and respiration taken 30 minutes after preanesthetic medication Pulse:			
Resp:			
10. Morning T.P.R. charted			
11. Operative permit signed and on chart			
12. Blood report on chart			
13. Urine report on chart			
14. Doctor's order sheet on chart			
15. Identification wristlet applied			
16. Colored nail polish removed (from at least 2 fingers)			

Signature of Nurse:_____

Date:_____

Fig. 57. Preoperative checklist, which is attached to the patient's chart and is checked immediately before the patient is taken to the operating room. (Also Fig. 77.)

Fig. 58. A ring secured to the finger with a bandage. (Sutton, A. L.: Bedside Nursing Techniques, p. 107, Philadelphia, Saunders, 1964)

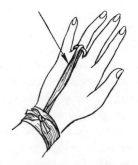

TRANSPORTATION OF THE PATIENT TO THE OPERATING ROOM

The patient is transported to the operating room in his own bed or a previously prepared stretcher. A small pillow may support his head. Top covers are tucked in at the sides and the foot of the stretcher; a wide strap is fastened in about the midthigh position to help keep the patient secure on the table. The covers should be adequate to protect the patient from exposure and chilling in draughty corridors. The conveyance is moved with the foot end proceeding first. The nurse remains at the head of the patient. When a stretcher has one pair of movable and one pair of fixed wheels, the patient's head is placed at the stationary end. If the patient is receiving intravenous fluids from a glass flask, caution should be taken that in the event of accidental breakage the flask is kept away from the patient's face. The chart accompanies the patient but should not be available to him; it is given to the anesthetist. Under no circumstances is the preoperative patient to be left unattended. He is taken to the anesthesia or the waiting room where it is quiet and darkened.

RECEPTION OF THE PATIENT IN THE OPERATING ROOM

The patient is greeted by the anesthetist or the nurse and made to feel that he is in secure hands. If he is to wait a few minutes, it must be in a quiet area away from traffic. He should not be left where he can see or hear undesirable sights or sounds from other patients or be disturbed by conversation of personnel that might be exaggerated, misinterpreted or in poor taste. Even when a patient appears to be drowsy and unconcerned, he may be acutely aware of sounds and voices. Finesse should be displayed by everyone in attendance. Skill in communication is conveyed not only by words but also by facial expression, manner, a reassuring touch or a warm grasp of the hand.

ANESTHESIA

Anesthesia is administered and controlled solely by professional personnel who have been trained in this highly complex and specialized science. As those who assist in surgery increase their understanding of anesthesia, they become more valuable members of the team working with the anesthesiologist and the surgeon.

CLASSIFICATION

An *anesthetic agent* is one that renders the patient insensible to pain, with or without loss of consciousness. Such an agent usually is administered by an anesthetist who is especially trained. The physician-anesthetist, whose field of study and practice involves the physiological changes of the body caused by anesthetics, is referred to as an *anesthesiologist*.

Anesthesia may be *general* (with loss of consciousness) or *local* (without loss of consciousness). General anesthesia affects the whole body. Agents which produce this may be administered (1) by inhalation, (2) intravenously or (3) rectally. Local anesthesia affects only a part of the body, and agents which produce this may be injected in (1) a local area, (2) a regional area or (3) the spinal canal.

CHOICE OF ANESTHETIC AGENT

This is usually made by the anesthesiologist in collaboration with the surgeon. Many factors affect the decision, such as the patient's age, condition and stature; the nature and the length of the operation; and the possibility of using explosive hazards such as cautery. When possible, the patient's preference may determine the choice of anesthetic drug.

STAGES OF GENERAL ANESTHESIA

Generally, anesthesia is described as having 4 stages. They are described in detail in Table 1, page 142. (See also Fig. 59.)

METHODS OF ADMINISTRATION

Inhalation. The anesthetic is inhaled and carried into the blood stream through the alveolar membranes in the lung. The nature of the agent and the depth of respirations determine the rapidity and the depth of anesthesia.

Technics for Administration are:

1. *Open-Drop.* The volatile liquid is dropped slowly on several layers of gauze held over the patient's nose and mouth (Fig. 60). The patient inhales the vapor and exhales through the gauze. The skin area around the mouth and the nose sometimes is lubricated to prevent skin irritation. Caution is taken to prevent a drop of the anesthetic from entering the eye.

2. *Vapor or Gas Administration With Mask.* Vapor from a liquid often is administered to the patient in combination with air, oxygen or a gas anesthetic. This is conducted to the patient by a tube and a mask. The gases (oxygen, nitrous oxide, ethylene and cyclopropane) are contained in tanks under pressure. By regulating valves the desired gases are conducted into a mixing chamber and then into a large rubber rebreathing bag. This is connected by a flexible corrugated tube to a mask, which is fastened over the nose and the mouth of the patient. The system used may

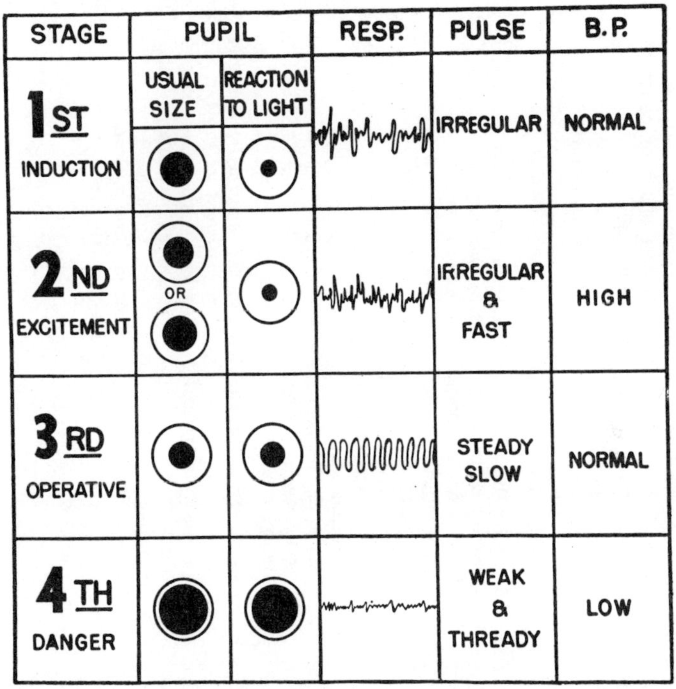

STAGE	PUPIL		RESP.	PULSE	B.P.
	USUAL SIZE	REACTION TO LIGHT			
1ST INDUCTION	◉	⊙		IRREGULAR	NORMAL
2ND EXCITEMENT	◉ OR ◉	⊙		IRREGULAR & FAST	HIGH
3RD OPERATIVE	⊙	⊙		STEADY SLOW	NORMAL
4TH DANGER	⬤	⬤		WEAK & THREADY	LOW

Fig. 59. Stages of anesthesia. (U.S. Army Manual, TM 8-230, Medical and Surgical Technicians)

Fig. 60. Technic of open-drop anesthesia. (A) Anesthetist dropping a volatile liquid anesthetic agent. (B) Cork out and wick in place to drip liquid agent. (Dripps, R. D., et al.: Introduction to Anesthesia, ed. 2, p. 87, Fig. 25, Philadelphia, Saunders, 1961)

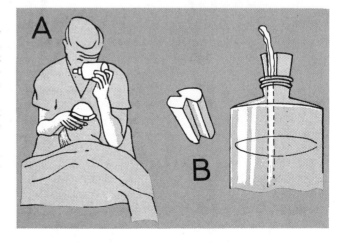

TABLE 1. STAGES OF ANESTHESIA

STAGE	PLANE	BIOLOGIC RESPONSE	DURATION	REACTION OF PATIENT	RESPONSIBILITY OF ATTENDANT TO THE ANESTHETIST
1. Induction	1	No analgesia No amnesia	From beginning of administration of anesthetic to loss of consciousness	Drowsy Dizzy Exaggerated hearing and feeling	*Keep room quiet* (the sense of hearing is the last phase of consciousness to leave the patient).
	2	Partial analgesia Total amnesia			*Stand at patient's side.*
	3	Total analgesia Total amnesia			
2. Excitement		Delirium	From loss of consciousness to relaxation	Irregular breathing Dreamy; delirious May be excited, vomit, hold breath or struggle May move extremities Highly susceptible to external stimuli such as being touched, a sudden noise, etc.	*Restrain patient if necessary.* *Assist anesthetist.* *Maintain quiet.*
3. Relaxation (surgical anesthesia)	1	Partial sensory loss	Relaxation to loss of reflexes	Quiet regular breathing	*Until the anesthetist has given permission, the assistant refrains from touching the patient. This could trigger a violent reaction of excitement if the patient is not "deep" enough.*
	2	Complete sensory loss		Fair muscular relaxation	*Then position patient.*
	3	Progressive intercostal paralysis		Insensible Relaxed jaw	*Prepare skin area for incision.*
	4	Complete intercostal paralysis			
4. Danger		Medullary paralysis Respiratory failure, possible cardiac arrest	Loss of reflexes to death	Breathing rapid and shallow Pulse rapid and thready Breathing stops.	*Assist in treatment for cardiac arrest and respiratory failure;* see pages, 253, 254; 257–261.

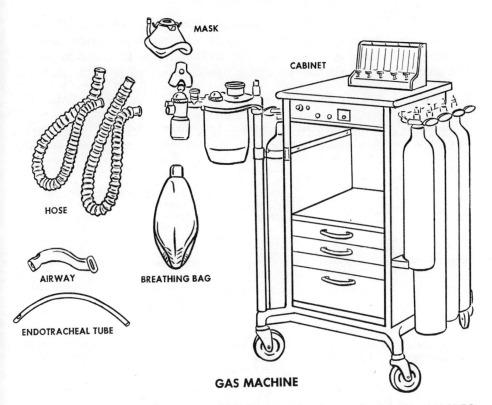

Fig. 61. Gas machine and pieces of equipment used by the anesthesiologist. (AMSCO, American Sterilizer Company, Erie, Pa.; Gibbons, C. P.: Care of anesthesia equipment, Hosp. Topics 42:110, September 1964)

be open, partially open or closed. The *open or nonrebreathing* method allows the patient to inhale only the anesthetic mixture delivered by the anesthetic machine. He exhales directly into the surrounding air. The *semiopen* system allows a portion of the exhaled gases to go out into the surrounding air and the remainder to be rebreathed. The *closed* type requires complete rebreathing of expired gases. In this system exhaled carbon dioxide is absorbed chemically, and oxygen as needed is delivered to the patient. Obviously, the last method reduces the problem of explosion and odors; less gas is wasted, thereby reducing cost. (Fig. 61)

3. *Insufflation.* Anesthetic gases and volatile liquids are delivered or blown into the upper respiratory passages by compressed air.

4. *Endotracheal.* Gases and volatile liquids are delivered through a soft rubber or plastic tube introduced directly into the trachea either "blindly" or by means of a laryngoscope.

GENERAL ANESTHETIC AGENTS

The search for the perfect anesthetic continues. Meanwhile, those in use provide a choice of method for administration, and each has its specific advantages and disadvantages. To achieve optimum effect, the anesthetist must be skilled in the use of the anesthetic and select the best one or combinations that fit the needs of the

TABLE 2. VOLATILE LIQUIDS AS AGENTS OF GENERAL ANESTHESIA

AGENT	ADMINISTRATION	ADVANTAGES	DISADVANTAGES	IMPLICATIONS
1. Ethyl ether	Open-drop; inhalation	Excellent relaxant Wide margin of safety Inexpensive Relatively non-toxic Used for all types of surgery	Slow induction: 10 minutes Long recovery; not eliminated for approximately 8 hours Irritating to skin, eyes, and kidneys May cause acidosis Causes nausea and vomiting Flammable and explosive	*Protect skin with lubricant.* *Instill sterile oil in eyes.* *Expect nausea and vomiting— turn head to side to prevent aspiration of vomitus.* *Practice safeguards in view of flammability.*
2. Vinyl ether (Vinethene)	Open-drop; inhalation	Induction very rapid Little postoperative vomiting Good for short procedures	Small margin of safety because of rapidity with which it acts May cause liver or kidney damage Increases salivation Flammable and explosive	*Protect skin and eyes to prevent irritation.* *Employ safeguards because of flammability.*
3. Halothane (Fluothane)	Inhalation; special vaporizers	Not explosive or inflammable Induction rapid and smooth Useful in almost every type of surgery Low incidence of postoperative nausea and vomiting	Expensive Requires skillful administration to prevent overdosage Has caused liver damage in a few cases May produce hypotension (low blood pressure) Requires special vaporizer for administration	*In addition to observing pulse and respiration postoperatively, it is important that blood pressure be determined frequently.*

AGENT	ADMINISTRATION	ADVANTAGES	DISADVANTAGES	IMPLICATIONS
4. Methoxy-flurane (Penthrane)	Inhalation; special vaporizer	Nonflammable; Nonexplosive Seldom causes postoperative nausea and vomiting Analgesic action continues several hours after surgery. Excellent muscle relaxation	Requires skillful administration	*Prolonged postoperative depressant action calls for careful observation by recovery room personnel.*

TABLE 3. GASES AS AGENTS OF GENERAL ANESTHESIA

AGENT	ADMINISTRATION	ADVANTAGES	DISADVANTAGES	IMPLICATIONS
1. Nitrous oxide (N_2O)	Inhalation (closed method)	Induction and recovery rapid Nonflammable Nonexplosive Useful with oxygen for short procedures Useful with other agents for all types of surgery	Poor relaxant Weak anesthetic May produce hypoxia	*Most useful in conjunction with other agents*
2. Cyclopropane (C_3H_6)	Inhalation (closed method)	Good relaxant Useful in all types of surgery Low toxicity	Explosive Expensive Powerful depressant; therefore should be administered skillfully Occasionally produces disturbances in heart rhythm May cause bronchospasm	*Employ precautions against explosions.* Because cyclopropane is a cardiac irritant, and the development of shock is a postoperative possibility, *it is important to observe blood pressure.* This usually is anticipated by the anesthetist, who administers Wyamine, a blood pressure elevator.

TABLE 4. INTRAVENOUS BARBITURATE AS AN AGENT OF GENERAL ANESTHESIA

AGENT	ADMINISTRATION	ADVANTAGES	DISADVANTAGES	IMPLICATIONS
Thiopental (Pentothal Sodium)	Intravenous injection	Rapid induction Nonexplosive Requires little equipment Low incidence of postoperative nausea and vomiting	Powerful depressant of breathing Poor relaxant Sometimes produces coughing and choking Not useful for children because of small veins	*Requires intelligent and close observation because of rapidity of drug action*

TABLE 5. RECTAL BASAL ANESTHETIC

AGENT	ADMINISTRATION	ADVANTAGES	DISADVANTAGES	IMPLICATIONS
1. Avertin	Rectally Amount of drug is calculated according to patient's weight.	Rapid action Can be administered in patient's unit; hence allays fears Used as supplement to other anesthetic agents	Marked respiratory depressant Throat reflexes depressed Poor relaxant	*Requires close observation for respiratory complications*
2. Pentothal rectal suspension	As above	Useful in children	As above	As above

individual patient. The following tables on the more common general anesthetics supply the method of administration, advantages and disadvantages, as well as implications.

LOCAL ANESTHESIA

Local anesthesia interrupts the normal passage of pain impulses from a certain area. It also depresses the superficial nerves.

Methods of Administration.

1. *Topical Anesthesia.* The anesthetic agent is applied directly to the site by being sprayed, as with ethylene chloride, by gentle rubbing, as with Nupercainal Ointment, or by application with a gauze pledget.

2. *Local or Infiltration Anesthesia.* A solution containing the local anesthetic drug is injected into the tissues through which the incision is to pass.

3. *Regional.* The anesthetic agent is injected in and around a particular nerve or group of nerves. This depresses sensation in a prescribed area supplied by these nerve trunks.

Of the nerve fibers, the motor fibers are the largest and have the thickest sheaths. Sensory fibers are intermediary in size, whereas autonomic or sympathetic fibers are the smallest, with a minimal covering. A local anesthetic blocks the motor nerves least readily. An anesthetic cannot be considered to be "worn off" until all three systems, motor, sensory and autonomic, are no longer affected by the agent.

Types of Regional Anesthesia. These are:

Nerve Block. Injection of a particular nerve.

Field Block. Production of prescribed field of anesthesia by several injections in and around the operative site. An example is paravertebral block.

Spinal. This is described later on page 149.

Caudal. Injection of the anesthetic agent epidurally through the caudal canal. This produces anesthesia of the perineum and, occasionally, the abdominal wall and the viscera. It is used in obstetrics.

METHODS OF INJECTION

I.M.—intramuscular—injected directly into muscle

I.V.—intravenous—injected directly into a vein

Subcut.—subcutaneous—injected just under the skin

EFFECTS ON BLOOD VESSELS

Vasoconstriction—reduces the size of the vessel

Vasodilatation—enlarges the size of the vessel

Advantages, Precautions and Disadvantages. Local anesthesia is popular for several reasons:

1. It is simple to use, economical, nonexplosive.
2. The required equipment is minimal.
3. Postoperative care is lessened.
4. It is ideal for short and superficial operations.

Local anesthesia is undesirable if the area requires many injections, as in a radical mastectomy. It should not be used in individuals who are apprehensive and highly nervous. In some instances patients may be sensitive to a local drug. If the patient is to receive the safest and most desired effects from these drugs, certain precautions should be observed:

1. Ask the patient whether he knows of any sensitivity to local anesthetics. The anesthetist may test the patient for sensitivity.

2. Provide fresh and sterile solutions. Frequently, drugs (colorless in appearance) come in glass ampules which must be accompanied by an ampule file. The label must be read carefully by the person providing the ampule as well as by the user. If the label is not legible, the ampule should be discarded. Most ampules today can be autoclaved safely. Those which are disinfected in a chemical should be kept in a tinted chemical; if there is a crack in the glass ampule, the tinted chemical can be detected in the ampule. This defective ampule should be discarded.

3. Observe the patient for reactions. Report them to the person administering the local anesthetic; in all likelihood he will stop giving the medication.

TABLE 6. LOCAL ANESTHETIC AGENTS

AGENT	ADMINISTRATION AND ACTION	ADVANTAGES	DISADVANTAGES	IMPLICATIONS
1. Cocaine (white crystalline powder readily soluble in water)	*Only* used *topically* Produces temporary paralysis of sensory nerve fibers Pulse elevated Respiration elevated	Rapid Patient is awake and can cooperate.	Possible idiosyncrasy (susceptibility) Possible addiction COCAINE REACTION 1. Exhilaration Excited Talkative Flushed face Muscular twitchings Rapid pulse 2. Shock Pallor Cyanosis Dilated pupils Apprehension Dyspnea Chills *Treatment:* Stop drug Oxygen Trendelenburg position Artificial respiration	*Never to be injected because of high toxicity* *Watch patient for reaction.* *If reaction, stay with patient and reassure him.* *Assist physician.*
2. Procaine (Novocain)	Solution, ½, 1, or 2% Subcut., I.M., I.V. or spinal	Low toxicity Inexpensive	Some idiosyncrasy (possibly skin flushing, increased pulse)	*Usually given with epinephrine.* This causes vasoconstriction, thereby slowing absorption and prolonging nerve-deadening effect.
3. Lidocaine (Xylocaine) and mepivacaine (Carbocaine)	Topical or injection	Rapid Longer duration of action (compared with procaine) Free from local irritative effect	Occasional idiosyncrasy Tends to spread from injection site	*Useful topically for cystoscopy* *Injected for use in dental work and surgery*

SPINAL ANESTHESIA

Anesthesia of the lower extremities, the abdomen and lateral kidney area may be induced by the introduction of drugs into a particular space in the spinal canal. This is a sterile procedure in which the patient usually is placed on his side (Fig. 62) with his knees drawn up to his stomach and his head bent forward. This position increases the spaces between the spinal vertebrae, making it easier for the anesthetist to insert a needle between the 3rd and the 4th lumbar vertebrae. The assistant can help the patient to maintain this position by holding the patient's knees up and the head down. At first a local anesthetic is administered to the selected lumbar area, and then the anesthesiologist inserts the spinal needle, usually a No. 22 with stylet in place. When he feels that he has pierced the dura (one of the meninges or coverings of the spinal canal), he withdraws the stylet, notes the trickling of spinal fluid and injects the required amount of local anesthetic. The patient then is turned to his back and positioned when the anesthesiologist assents.

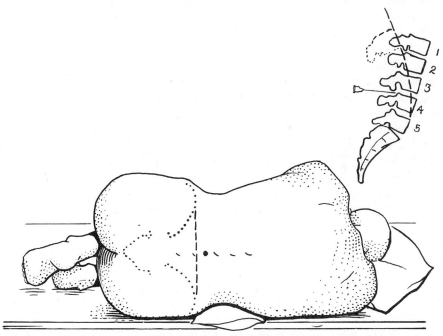

Fig. 62. Lateral position for the administration of spinal anesthesia. Note that the needle is inserted between the 3rd and the 4th lumbar vertebra. (Brunner, L. S., et al.: Textbook of Medical-Surgical Nursing, p. 909, Philadelphia, Lippincott, 1964)

TABLE 7. SPINAL ANESTHESIA

AGENTS	ADVANTAGES OF SPINAL ANESTHESIA (Includes All Agents)	DISADVANTAGES OF SPINAL ANESTHESIA (Includes All Agents)
Procaine (Novocain) Tetracaine (Pontocaine) Dibucaine (Nupercaine)	Easily administered by a physician Inexpensive Minimum of equipment required Rapid onset Excellent muscular relaxation	Blood pressure may fall rapidly unless watched carefully and treated with such drugs as ephedrine, etc. If the spinal anesthesia ascends to the chest, there may be respiratory difficulties. Occasionally, postoperative complications occur, such as headache, paralysis or meningitis.

ANESTHETIC AIDS

DRUGS

Preanesthetic medications have been discussed on page 137.

Muscle Relaxants. When these drugs are given in carefully controlled doses, lighter anesthesia can be used, thereby reducing the hazards inherent in deep anesthesia.

The original muscle relaxant, curare,* had dangerous side-effects which stimulated chemists to attempt to synthesize new compounds with safer muscle-relaxing properties. Today the anesthetist has a considerable array of drugs available for bringing about almost any desired degree of relaxation. Syncurine, Metubine and Anectine are examples of curarelike synthetic drugs. All must be administered carefully by a skilled anesthesiologist, since there is a narrow margin between safe dosage and overdosage. A distinctive label should be placed on the intravenous bottle when a muscle relaxant is given by infusion. If too much relaxation occurs, the respiratory muscles may become paralyzed. Fortunately, there are antagonist drugs which counteract the effects of muscle relaxants. An example of such a drug is neostigmine (Prostigmin).

THE OPERATING TABLE

Most operating tables consist of a rectangular metal top that rests on a hydraulic or a motorized wheeled base. The tabletop is divided into 3 or 5 hinged sections, all of which can be moved individually or elevated by means of a control. Flexing or extending the table is often referred to as "breaking" the table. Nurses and technicians must be familiar with the operation of tables and their attachments. Any desirable position of the patient can be achieved when he is placed on the

* Curare has been used by South American Indians for centuries as a poison for their arrows. This poison, which is obtained from a plant, causes death by paralyzing the respiratory muscles.

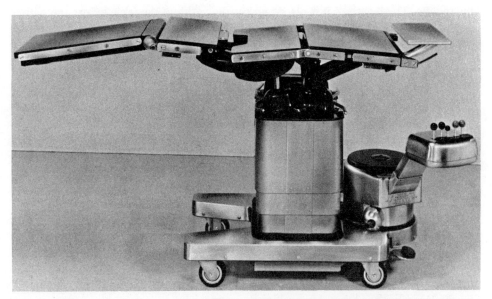

Fig. 63. Operating table. (Wilmot Castle Company, Rochester, N.Y.)

operating table, provided that the individual knows (1) how to operate the table, (2) what position the surgeon desires, (3) how to adjust the table to meet the anatomic needs of the particular patient and (4) how to maintain this position for the duration of the operation. (Fig. 63)

The entire table can be tilted from side to side, raised and lowered, and the foot and the head ends can be elevated or lowered. A tiltmeter indicates the degree of tilt that is helpful to the anesthetist when spinal anesthesia is administered. A brake locks the table in position.

ATTACHMENTS AND EQUIPMENT FOR THE OPERATING TABLE

Attachments are provided to assist in maintaining the desired position of the patient on the table. Such pieces of equipment should be padded to prevent injury.

The body restraint strap is a wide leather or heavy canvas strap, sometimes covered with conductive material, that is fastened with a buckle. This strap is applied as soon as the patient is placed on the operating table and is kept in place above the knees for all dorsal positions. It must be applied securely and yet not hinder circulation.

The anesthesia screen is a metal rod which holds the sterile drapes up and off the face of the patient, thereby providing an area of freedom for the anesthetist to care for and observe the patient.

The arm holder (drawsheet or patient lifter) is a width of heavy muslin approximately 2 yards long by 15 inches wide (Fig. 64). It is double and stitched through the middle. The length of it is placed across the width of the table before the patient is placed on top of it. Each of the two ends is rolled around the patient's arms in opposite turns as shown in Figure 64. This serves as an arm restraint. Later this is a convenient holder for those assisting in moving the patient to his bed or recovery room stretcher.

Padded leather wristlets also can be used to keep the arms at the side. These often are part of the operating table.

The armboard, which may be wooden or metal (covered with conductive sheeting), may be used to support the arm when an intravenous infusion is given, or when it is necessary to provide a support for the arm. During hand or arm surgery the armboard serves as an extended operating table.

Padded body and kidney rests are devices to stabilize the body in certain necessary positions for nephrectomy or biliary surgery.

The footboard is a metal board placed at the foot of the table to provide support for the feet of the patient as they rest against it. It is particularly desirable in reverse Trendelenburg position.

Stirrups or lithotomy leg holders are metal posts that can be fastened in place to the side rail near the lower segment of the table. These provide the means of support for the legs when the lithotomy position is desired.

Pillows and sandbags also are available to provide additional means of support and security for the patient.

POSITIONING THE PATIENT

PREPARATION

The anesthetist indicates when the patient can be moved to the desired position. The nurse or the technician has available the necessary equipment and sufficient help to position the patient skillfully. He should be moved with proper regard for normal body movement; relaxed extremities need support to prevent dangling or getting caught. The anesthetist usually is responsible for supporting and turning the head. Unnecessary exposure of the patient is avoided.

POSITIONING THE PATIENT FOR SURGERY

The position to be assumed by a patient for the duration of the operative procedure is determined by many requirements.

A good position must provide:

1. The best possible exposure and accessibility of the operative field for the surgeon.

2. The best possible access to the patient for the administration of the anesthetic agent and the observation of its effects on the patient.

3. Access for the administration of intravenous solutions.

4. Comfort and safety for the patient.

The patient is positioned by the circulating nurse and her assistant, or the anesthetist, or the surgeon or his assistants, depending on the local hospital procedure. This may vary with individual circumstances. Usually, the patient is positioned after the administration of the general anesthetic when the anesthetist permits. For local anesthesia the patient is positioned prior to injection.

Principles to be observed in positioning the patient for surgery are as follows:

1. *Proper respiratory functioning should be maintained.* The jaw should be forward and not allowed to drop on the chest, thereby shutting off the airway. Constriction of or pressure on the chest should be avoided to permit free exchange of gases. The gown should not constrict the neck.

2. *Unimpaired circulation must be insured.* Avoid pressure on any part of the body, particularly the extremities, which would interfere with venous flow of blood. In the lateral (side-lying) position, the upper leg could exert pressure on the lower leg, thus hindering circulation, unless a soft pillow separates the legs. Straps or adhesive tape used to fix the extremities must not be applied too tightly.

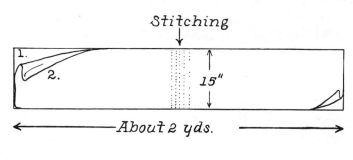

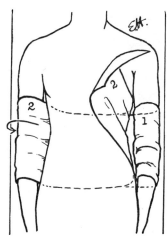

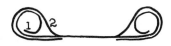

Fig. 64. Combination arm holder and body lift for use on operating table. (Brunner, L. S., *et al.:* Textbook of Medical-Surgical Nursing, p. 230, Philadelphia, Lippincott, 1964)

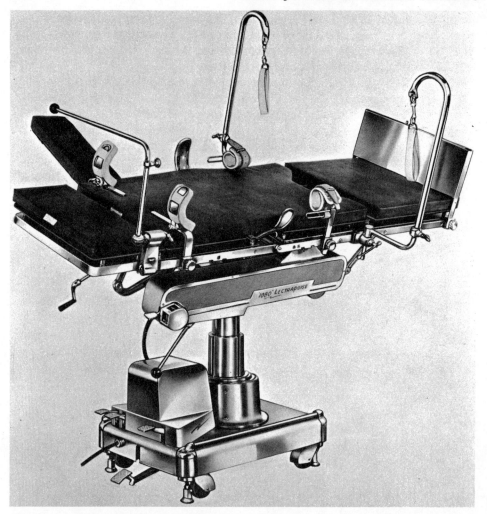

Fig. 65. Lectrapoise surgical table showing attachments in place. (AMSCO, American Sterilizer Company)

3. *Muscles and nerves must be protected from undue pressure.* Everyone is familiar with the sensation of a limb's "going to sleep" following nerve pressure such as that caused by prolonged crossing of the legs. Improper positioning of the extremities may cause serious injury or paralysis (Fig. 66). In Trendelenburg position, for example, the shoulder braces must be well padded to prevent irreparable nerve damage (Figs. 68, 70). By using a soft pad under the knee, injury to the popliteal nerve is prevented.

4. *Concern for the patient as an individual must be practiced.* Very thin, elderly or obese patients need particular attention to prevent respiratory, circulatory and

nerve difficulties. The emotional state as well as the dignity of the individual patient must be considered by those in attendance. Undue exposure of the patient should be avoided.

Common Operative Positions. These are:

Dorsal Recumbent. The usual position is flat on the back with the arms at the side of the table, palms down (Fig. 69, *top*). Legs are straight. This position is used for abdominal operations.

Modified Dorsal Recumbent. This is similar to the above position with the

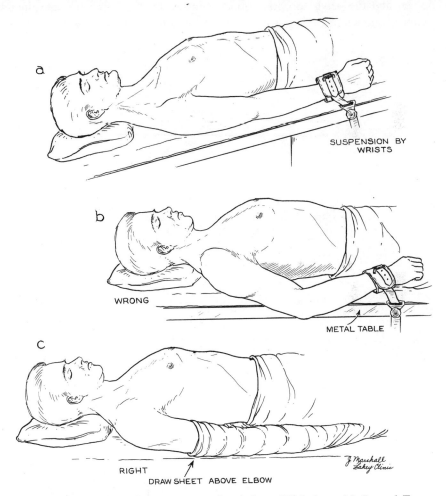

Fig. 66. Dangers from improper use of wristlets. (Nicholson, M. J., and Ever-sole, U. H.: Nerve injuries incident to anesthesia and operation *in* Surgical Practice of the Lahey Clinic, Philadelphia, Saunders, 1962, and there a revision of an article published in Anesthesia and Analgesia 36:19–32, 1957)

exception that the knees are slightly flexed with a pillow underneath, and the thighs are rotated externally. This position is used for saphenous ligations and groin operations.

Dorsal Recumbent With Arm Extension. The patient is flat, and the legs are straight. The arm on the affected side is on an armboard at a not-greater-than 90° angle from the body. This position is desired in mastectomy and hand surgery (Figs. 68, 69, *bottom*). Note pillow supports.

Trendelenburg Position. This position usually is used for operations on the lower abdomen and the pelvis to obtain good exposure by displacing the intestines into the upper abdomen. In this position the head and the body are lowered. The knees

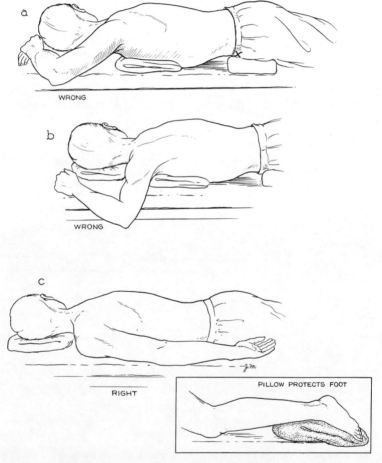

Fig. 67. Prone position, right and wrong (Nicholson, M. J., and Eversole, U. H.: Nerve injuries incident to anesthesia and operation *in* Surgical Practice of the Lahey Clinic, Philadelphia, Saunders, 1962, and there a revision of an article published in Anesthesia and Analgesia 36:19–32, 1957)

are flexed by "breaking" the table, and the patient is held in position by padded shoulder braces. (Fig. 70)

This position is slightly modified for the patient who is going into shock. In this condition, usually the foot end is not flexed, but the table is kept straight with the head low and the feet elevated.

Prone Position. The patient is lying on his abdomen. Proper supports are placed, as indicated in Figure 67. This position is used for operations on the spine and the posterior chest.

Lithotomy Position. The patient is on his back. When he is under the influence

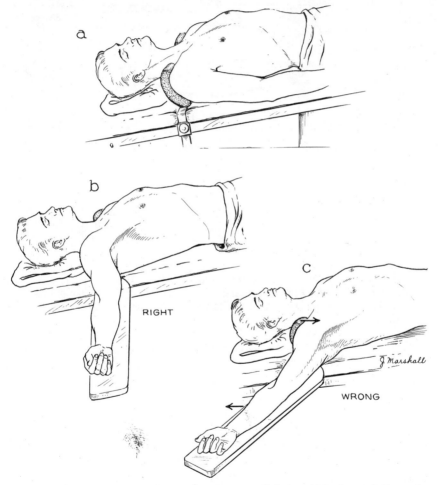

Fig. 68. Shoulder braces, right and wrong. (Nicholson, M. J., and Eversole, U. H.: Nerve injuries incident to anesthesia and operation *in* Surgical Practice of the Lahey Clinic, Philadelphia, Saunders, 1962, and there a revision of an article published in Anesthesia and Analgesia 36:19–32, 1957)

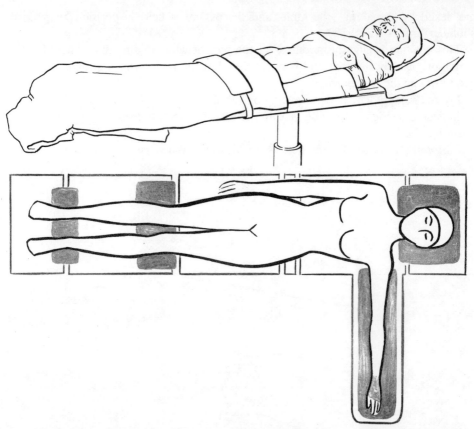

Fig. 69. Patient in position on the operating table as prepared for a laparotomy. Note the
strap above the knees and the arm holder in use. (*Top,* Brunner, L. S., *et al.:*
Textbook of Medical-Surgical Nursing, p. 232, Fig. 49 A, Philadelphia, Lippincott, 1964; *bottom,* Davis & Geck, Division of American Cyanamid Company,
Danbury, Conn.)

of anesthesia, the thighs and the legs are flexed to right angles. If stirrups are
attached to metal posts, the legs are placed on the outside of the posts, and the
ankles and the feet are supported by canvas straps (Fig. 71). Some operating
tables have metal angular supports on which the flexed leg is supported. In this
position the buttocks are placed at the table edge with the lowermost portion of the
table lowered. Perineal, rectal and vaginal operations require this position. It is
desirable that both legs be positioned at the same time. Likewise, in returning the
patient to the dorsal position, both legs are removed from the supports simultaneously and slowly moved to the flat position.

Kidney Position. After the patient is anesthetized, he is placed on the unaffected
side with his back near the edge of the table (Fig. 72). He is also placed so that
the kidney area is directly above the body elevator. This position is used for kidney
and ureter surgery.

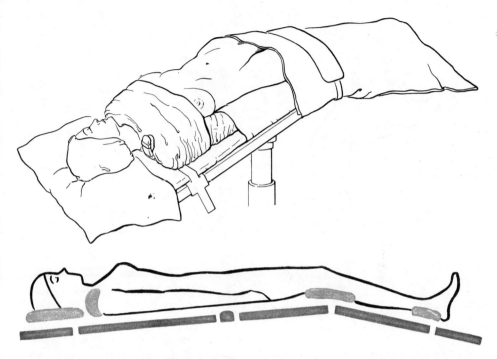

Fig. 70. Patient in Trendelenburg position on operating table. Note padded shoulder braces in place. (*Top,* Brunner, L. S., *et al.:* Textbook of Medical-Surgical Nursing, p. 232, Fig. 49 B, Philadelphia, Lippincott, 1964; *bottom,* Davis & Geck, Division of American Cyanamid Company)

Thoracic Surgery. The position varies with the operation to be performed. This is affected by the nature of the incision, the optimum exposure, the type of anesthesia and the surgeon's preference.

For thyroid or neck surgery the patient is on his back with the neck somewhat extended by a pillow beneath the shoulders.

For brain and bone surgery a special operating table usually is used, which is adjusted by the surgeon.

PREPARATION OF THE OPERATIVE AREA

Removal of hair and cleansing of skin around the operative site have been discussed on page 133. Following the positioning of the patient on the operating table, the lights are adjusted and focused, and the table is locked in position. The area of operation is generously exposed. As a rule, a cleansing scrub of this area is done in the operating room which is generally more thorough than that which accompanied the preoperative shave. The assistant to the surgeon or a nurse prepares the skin with antiseptic. Sterile gloves are worn by this person, and he uses gauze pledgets or a sponge forceps which holds the "prep" gauze. The choice

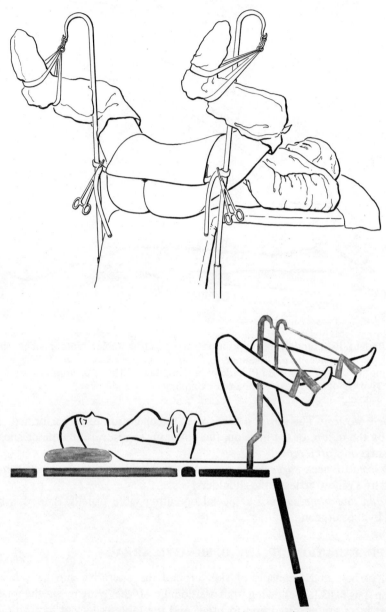

Fig. 71. Patient in lithotomy position. Note that the hips extend over the edge of the table. (*Top,* Brunner, L. S., *et al.*: Textbook of Medical-Surgical Nursing, p. 232, Fig. 49 C, Philadelphia, Lippincott, 1964; *bottom,* Davis & Geck, Division of American Cyanamid Company)

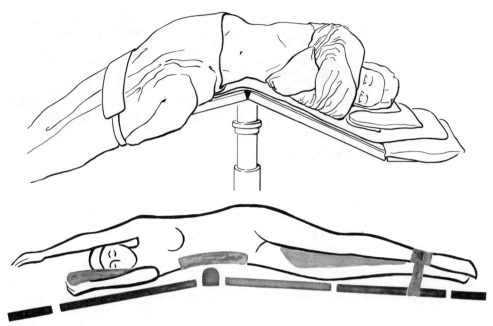

Fig. 72. Patient on operating table for kidney operation, lying on his well side. Table is broken to spread apart space between the lower ribs and the pelvis. The upper leg is extended; the lower leg is flexed at the knee and the hip joints; a pillow is placed between the legs. Note the sandbag, which helps to support the patient's chest. (*Top,* Brunner, L. S., *et al.:* Textbook of Medical-Surgical Nursing, p. 232, Fig. 49 D, Philadelphia, Lippincott, 1964; *bottom,* Davis & Geck, Division of American Cyanamid Company)

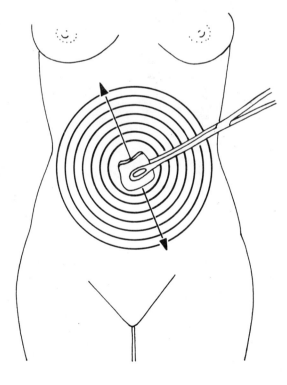

Fig. 73. Start abdominal "prep" at site of incision. Move outward in circular motion. Do not return sponge to center but discard. (Nursing Care of the Patient in Ob-Gyn Surgery, p. 30, Fig. 33, Somerville, N.J., Ethicon, Inc.)

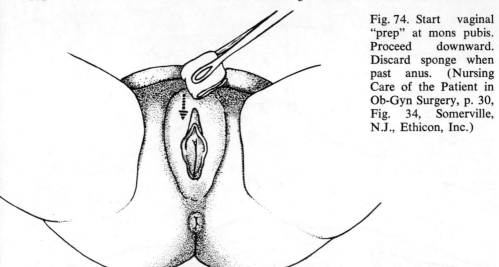

Fig. 74. Start vaginal "prep" at mons pubis. Proceed downward. Discard sponge when past anus. (Nursing Care of the Patient in Ob-Gyn Surgery, p. 30, Fig. 34, Somerville, N.J., Ethicon, Inc.)

of antiseptics usually is determined by the surgeon. The incision line is painted first, and the antiseptic is applied to increasingly larger areas, working outward to the periphery (this displaces microorganisms away from the operative site). The sponge is discarded, and a new one is used to repeat the process (Fig. 73). A

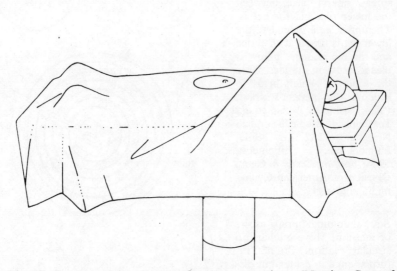

Fig. 75. Fenestrated laparotomy sheet covers patient. (Nursing Care of the Patient in Ob-Gyn Surgery, p. 32, Fig. D, Somerville, N.J., Ethicon, Inc.)

sponge which has touched the edges of the prepared area is not used at the incision site because of the possibility of bringing bacteria to the cleanest area.

Some examples of effective skin antisepsis are the following:

1. Wash alternately with 70 per cent alcohol and tincture of Zephiran, each three times.

2. Apply acetone, and when the skin is dry, paint or preferably scrub with Ioprep.

3. Wet skin with water, apply Betadine surgical scrub* (1 cc. is sufficient to cover an area 20 to 30 sq. in.) and rub thoroughly for 5 minutes. Then develop a lather and rinse off by aid of sterile gauze saturated with water or blot with sterile towel and paint with Betadine antiseptic. (Also see p. 89, Chap. 6.)

Particular attention to the difficult areas such as the umbilicus must be given. Cotton-tipped applicators are useful. A check should be made of the area on which the patient is lying to be sure that he is not lying in a puddle. It may be necessary to use towels to soak up excess solution in order to prevent excoriation or burns of the skin.

The procedure for using antiseptic solution on other areas of the body may vary, depending on the nature of the site and the individual preference. For vaginal preparation, for example, external washing and internal cleansing are necessary. First the outer area is washed carefully, starting at the mons pubis and working downward (Fig. 74). The use of a sponge forceps with fresh sponges is necessary to clean the vagina thoroughly. Generous amounts of solutions are used, since there are many folds and crevices.

After the skin has been prepared, the patient is ready for draping.

PATIENT DRAPING

(See Drapes and Draping, p. 97.)

The patient is covered with drapes in such a way that only the operative site is exposed. Usually 4 towels are carefully placed and fastened to frame the incision site, or a self-adhering plastic is applied directly over this area. A fenestrated (having a window or hole) fanfolded laparotomy sheet is centered over the operative site and unfolded carefully outward (Fig. 75). The metal anesthesia screen holds the drapes away from the patient's face.

The draping of a patient in lithotomy position may be done by using the self-adhering plastic drape to cover the perineum and the surrounding area. When linens are used, a sterile sheet may be placed under the hips (Fig. 76) and a sterile towel used to cover the anus (shown secured by adhesive tape). Following these procedures a large sterile lithotomy sheet with leggings completes the draping by covering the legs and the body of the patient.

* Physicians Products Co., Petersburg, Virginia.

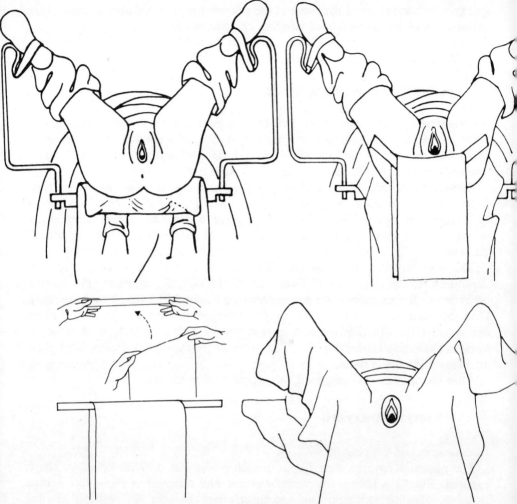

Fig. 76. A method of vaginal draping. (A) Sterile sheet is placed under hips. (B) Circulating nurse holds length of adhesive tape. (C) Scrub nurse places sterile towel over tape. (D) Circulating nurse secures tape to patient so that sterile towel covers anus. (E) Lithotomy sheet covers patient. (Nursing Care of the Patient in Ob-Gyn Surgery, p. 33, Figs. A, B, C, D, E, Somerville, N.J., Ethicon, Inc.)

REVIEW QUESTIONS:

1. Why is proper identification of a patient necessary? How is proper identification assured?
2. Under what conditions may a patient sign his own operative permit? What is done when a patient is unable to sign his operative permit?

3. Explain the action in general of hexachlorophene on the skin. Can alcohol be used on the skin after hexachlorophene? Why?
4. What precautions are used preoperatively in shaving the skin of a patient?
5. How would you apply a skin depilatory? What does it do?
6. List 3 categories of preanesthetic medications and explain the purpose of each.
7. Differentiate hypoxia from hypoxemia.
8. Why is stage 3 of general anesthesia more desirable than stages 2 and 4?
9. What are the responsibilities of the assistant during the induction of anesthesia?
10. What are the differences between the open and the closed systems in administering general anesthesia?
11. What precautions are taken in an operating room when an explosive gas such as cyclopropane is used?
12. What are the symptoms and the treatment of cocaine poisoning?
13. Describe the role of the assistant when a patient is to have spinal anesthesia.
14. Name two purposes of a muscle relaxant.
15. What principles must be followed in positioning a patient for surgery?
16. Differentiate between flexion and extension.
17. What precautions must be observed in placing a patient in lithotomy position?
18. How can the operative site be made as clean as possible during immediate preoperative preparation?
19. Describe and discuss the merits of the antiseptics used in your hospital as an abdominal skin "prep."
20. What principles should be observed in draping a patient? Could the method employed in your operating room be improved? How?

Bibliography

Breckenridge, F. J., and Bruno, P.: Nursing care of the anesthetized patient, Am. J. Nurs. 62:74–78, July 1962.
Dripps, R. D., Eckenhoff, J. E., and Vandam, L.: Introduction to Anesthesia, ed. 2, Philadelphia, Saunders, 1961.
Genereux, T. B.: Positioning patients in the operating room, Am. J. Nurs. 59:1572–1574, 1959.
Holt, M. B.: Hospital study of a depilatory cream for surgical patients, A.O.R.N.J. 2:66–71, March–April 1964.
Nicholson, M. J., and Eversole, U. H.: Nerve injuries incident to anesthesia and operation, A.O.R.N.J. 2:44–65, March–April 1964.

CHAPTER 9

PATIENT RECORDS

THE CHART : REQUISITES OF A GOOD CHART : KINDS OF RECORDS

THE CHART

From the time a patient is admitted to a hospital a written record is kept of everything pertaining to him and his condition. This record is known as the patient's *chart*. Although the types of records and the reasons for them may vary from one hospital to another, in all cases the aim is to develop charts that are informative and meaningful to the authorized personnel who will be using them throughout the patient's stay.

For example, on admission a list of the patient's clothes is made. Any valuables not taken by the patient's family are placed in the hospital safe, and a receipt is given. Accurate lists, signed by the nurse and the patient or his representative, are mandatory from a legal point of view.

A personal (sometimes called social) and a medical history are required and are recorded on the appropriate forms. A doctor's order sheet is used by the physician to record his instructions for the care of the patient; this includes all treatments, tests and medications. There are sheets for nurses' notes used by nurses to record treatments, medications and observations of the patient.

Depending on the disease or the condition of the patient, other sheets may be added to the routine chart to record the results of special tests, x-ray reports, pathologic reports and other pertinent information. In this manner all information about the patient, his care, diagnosis and treatment is in one place. Pertinent data, such as repeated laboratory tests, are so placed that comparisons can be made easily, and the response of the patient to treatment and medication is shown. Future plans and the progress of the patient make the chart a continuing and up-to-date record.

REQUISITES OF A GOOD CHART

If charts are to be useful, the writing must be legible and the information accurate and complete. To make the information more legible, many institutions prefer that charting or recording be done by printing rather than writing. Entries on charts are dated, signed or initialed (nurses' notes, etc.) or identified by the department with a signature (for instance, the x-ray interpretation is signed by the radiologist).

The information contained in a patient's chart is personal and confidential. No one is permitted to disclose chart information to unauthorized personnel without the consent of the patient. If disclosed, this constitutes a breach of ethics and is an infringement of the patient's right of privacy.

Operating room nursing personnel are concerned mainly with the sections of the chart that directly affect the surgical experience of the patient.

KINDS OF RECORDS

OPERATIVE PERMIT

An operative permit is a legal requirement prior to surgery. (See Chap. 8, p. 132.) This is sometimes called a signed surgical consent. The surgeon explains to the patient the surgical procedure anticipated and obtains his signed consent to undergo anesthesia and the specific surgical procedure. Ambiguously worded consent forms have been the cause of untold numbers of legal suits for malpractice, because the patient may have signed the form without knowing exactly what he was signing. Consent forms should not be signed as a routine part of the patient's admission to the hospital; nor should they be signed by the patient after sedation has been given.

The hospital policies governing this procedure (also approved by the Law Department of the American Medical Association[1]) usually state that if a patient is scheduled for and arrives in surgery after sedation without having properly signed a consent form, the surgery (except in an emergency) shall be cancelled and postponed until a properly signed form can be executed.

The signing of the operative permit is the responsibility of the surgeon. If it has not been done, the nurse can remind him that it must be. The physical examination and the history usually are done by internes or resident physicians. The laboratory work that has been ordered should be completed the day before, and the results recorded on the chart, because they may have direct bearing on the surgery planned.

PREOPERATIVE CHECKLIST

The preparation of a patient for surgery is important to the safety of a patient and his recovery from surgical experience. The preoperative checklist is used as a reminder to the personnel preparing him for surgery that the items listed must not be overlooked.

Checklists which include a section "Day Before Surgery" (sample, Fig. 77; also see Chap. 8, p. 137) are preferred by many.

[1] Medicolegal Forms With Legal Analysis, Chicago, Law Department, American Medical Association, 1961.

PREOPERATIVE CHECKLIST

	NURSES' INITIALS
Day Before Surgery:	
1. Operative permit has been signed	_____
2. History and Physical Exam on chart	_____
3. C.B.C. and Urinalysis on chart	_____
4. Consultation sheet signed and on chart as required by Hospital Policy	_____
5. Operative area prepared by	_____
6. Bleeding and Coagulation Time on chart of T and A Pts.	_____
7. Religion of patient is	_____
If Catholic, Priest has been notified of surgery	_____
Day of Surgery:	
1. Operative area checked by	_____
2. T.P.R. and B.P. are charted	_____
3. Voided or catheterized: Time and amount on chart	_____
4. Cosmetics, hairpins, dentures, jewelry removed	_____
5. Wedding band taped or tied	_____
6. Religious medals on gown	_____
7. Complete recheck of Doctor's preoperative orders	_____
8. Identification bracelet applied	_____
9. Pathology sheet on chart	_____
10. Completed preoperative check sheet:	_____

Signed by _____

Date _____

Fig. 77. (The Chester County Hospital, West Chester, Pa.)

Consultation sheets are required under some circumstances and must be signed and on the chart before the patient is in the operating room. Hospital policy dictates when consultation sheets are necessary.

The operative area is shaved and prepared, usually by operating room personnel. In some institutions ward personnel are assigned this duty. When the procedure has been completed by a responsible person, he or she signs the checklist in the space provided.

T & A (tonsillectomy and adenoidectomy) patients usually have blood testing done for clotting and bleeding. If the blood analysis proves to be abnormal, the surgery usually is postponed until normal limits are obtained.

Religious matters and notification of the clergy usually are handled by the family. However, if the patient or his family cannot do this, the nurse notifies the appropriate person, according to the hospital policy governing such circumstances. Many hospitals have chaplains who work with the nursing and the medical staffs to give spiritual assistance.

On the day of the scheduled operation the nurse responsible for the care of the patient that day checks the "Day of Surgery" part of the preoperative checklist.

Operative Site Check. The surface of the skin at the site of the incision must be free of hair and clean shaven. If it is not, it is necessary to redo the skin preparation before surgery. Checking this before the patient is in the operating room will save time and avoid anxiety after the patient is on the operating table.

T.P.R. and B.P. (temperature, pulse, respirations and blood pressure). Temperature and blood pressure are charted routinely for each surgery patient before the patient goes to the operating room. An elevated temperature or an abnormal pressure should be called to the attention of the surgeon and the anesthetist.

Voided or Catheterized. The bladder should be empty when the patient comes to the operating room. The time and the amount of the last voiding should be recorded.

Cosmetics, hairpins, dentures, jewelry, gum, etc., are removed (see Chap. 8, p. 137).

Doctor's Preoperative Orders. Orders must be carried out and so charted. If an error should occur, the surgeon should be notified immediately.

Identification Bracelet (see Chap. 8, p. 131). The bracelet should be in place on the patient's wrist or ankle.

Pathology Sheet on Chart. The specimen or specimens sent to the laboratory for examination are accompanied by a pathology request sheet signed by the physician. The operating room usually keeps extra request sheets for use when needed. The floor nurse is responsible for placing a pathology sheet on the chart of each patient going to surgery. The operating room personnel are responsible for sending this sheet, appropriately completed, with the specimen to the laboratory.

Completed Preoperative Check Sheet. When the preoperative checklist is completed, the floor nurse responsible for the preoperative care of the patient signs and dates it. It is then left on the chart to be given to the nurse receiving the patient in the operating room. The operating room nurse quickly can determine whether all of the items on the checklist have been completed and evaluate the significance of any notations for the operating room personnel.

LABORATORY REPORTS

The results of all laboratory work ordered and done before surgery must be on the chart when the patient comes to the operating room. Urinalysis, red and white blood cell counts, bleeding and coagulation time, and blood typing for transfusion are of vital importance to the surgeon in his care of the patient during the operation.

SPECIAL INFORMATION

Notification of allergies to drugs, sensitivity to chemical solutions or detergents, or other idiosyncrasies that the patient knows he has usually is affixed to the front of the chart with scotch tape in large attention-demanding letters. In some hospitals there are special red slips furnished for this purpose. A diabetic condition and information concerning times and dosages of insulin also might be in a prominent place on the front of the chart so that immediate attention is called to this fact by all personnel handling the patient.

OPERATING ROOM DATA SLIP
(Figs. 78, 79)

Operating Room Data Slips are filled out by the circulating nurse while the patient is in the operating room, and they usually are developed according to the needs of the individual surgery. The permanent records that are kept in surgery will determine the kinds of information that should be on the data slip. The circulating nurse fills out the heading (if an identification plate is used, space can be left at the top of each form to accommodate its print), the date, the name of the patient, the surgeon, the assistant or assistants, and the preoperative diagnosis. At the beginning of surgery, "time in" is recorded. "Anesthesia" and "anesthetist" also are noted, as are the names of the scrub assistant and the circulating nurse. The "operation" and "postoperative diagnosis" blanks should not be completed until the end of the operation, because in some instances these will differ from the preoperative diagnosis and the anticipated operation. The surgeon provides this information.

If the operation is a long one, and any of the assistants are relieved and replaced by other personnel, the names of all those participating should be recorded on the surgery data slip (example, Scrub Assistant: Layman/Smith). If two people are scrub assistants (often called 1st and 2nd scrub), both names are listed.

In some hospitals operating room charges are based on the length of time from the making of the incision to the closing of the wound. In these instances "time in" could mean 10 or 15 minutes after the start of anesthesia. Anesthesia charges,

SURGERY DATA SLIP

(patient's stamp)

File No._____ Rm. & Class_____

Date _____

Name _____

Surgeon _____

Assist. _____

Anesthesia _____

Anesthetist _____

Pre-Op Diag. _____

Post-Op Diag. _____

Operation _____
Scrub Assist.
   or Nurse _____

Cir. Nurse _____

Time In: _____ Out: _____

Charges _____

Fig. 78. Sample of a Surgery Data Slip. (Adapted from Surgery Data Slip, The Chester
County Hospital, West Chester, Pa.)

handled by the department of anesthesia, usually are calculated from the time the
anesthesia is started until the patient is removed from the operating room. In
other institutions flat charges or fees are made for certain types of surgery (i.e.,
major, minor, T & A, etc.), and time is not recorded.

A permanent record book of operations is kept in most operating room suites
for statistical purposes. In some hospitals this record is compiled in the medical
records department. In hospitals in which the former applies, the information from
the surgical data slips can be transferred directly to the book. Special patient
charges usually are billed by the business office. These may include blood, special
drugs, catheters or other special drainage tubing, prostheses and I.V. fluids.
Charge times are taken from the surgery data slips by a clerk or the ward secretary
and listed for patient charges.

DATA RECORD

Ward _____ Date _____

Patient _____ Age_____

Surgeon _____

Assist. Surgeon _____

Anesthetist _____

Scrub Nurse _____

Circulator _____

Anesthesia _____ Time Started_____ .

Operation _____

_____

Time Started _____ Ended _____

Charges: I.V., Drugs, Supplies_____

_____

_____

_____

Sponge Count_____

Preoperative Diagnosis _____

_____

Postoperative Diagnosis _____

_____

Remarks _____

_____

_____

_____

Fig. 79. Sample of a Surgery Data Sheet.

SPONGE COUNT RECORD

The purpose of the sponge count sheet is to help the personnel to keep an accurate account of the sponges used and to make the final count at the end of the case easier to tally. It becomes a part of the operating room records at the end of the surgery, and only the final result is recorded on the anesthetist's operative record sheet, which remains on the patient's chart. (Fig. 80)

SPONGE COUNT RECORD

Name _____   Date _____

Operation _____

Surgeon _____

No. 1

| Type | Beginning | Added | Total |

4 x 4

Pledgets

Long Sponge

No. 2

| Type | In Bag | On Chuck | Total |

4 x 4

Pledgets

Long Sponge

Remarks: _____

Subtract No. 2 Total from No. 1

4 x 4   _____

Pledgets   _____

Long Sponge   _____

1st. Sponge Count _____

2nd Sponge Count _____

_____
Circulating Nurse Signature

Fig. 80. Sponge Count Record. (Adapted from Sponge Count, The Chester County Hospital, West Chester, Pa.)

In the actual use of the Sponge Count sheet shown in Figure 80, the person who gives the scrub assistant added sponges during the progress of the case records the number and initials the entry. The lines are far enough apart to leave room for several entries if they are needed. In the event of a question of correct count, this practice makes it easier to pinpoint where an error might have been made.

Sponge counts are taken according to operating room policy and procedure. The method varies in institutions, but the desired result is the same, that is, accounting for all sponges used. In Figure 81 the physician counts the sponges he has in the field at the time the count is taken, but in some situations the scrub assistant also is responsible for this count.

Whatever the form adopted or the method used, a sponge count sheet is useful and necessary to help in keeping sponge counts accurate.

SPONGE COUNT

Doctor_____ Operation_____Date _____

	Raytec 4 x 8	Lg. Laps	Sm. Laps	Pushers
Case started with:				
Sponges Added				
Sponges Added				
Total Sponges to Scrub Nurse				
Circulating Nurse (discarded sponges)				
Scrub Nurse (on back table)				
Total				
Sponges needed: (in field)				
Doctor				
Total				

Signature _____

Fig. 81. Sample of a Sponge Count Record.

ANESTHESIA SHEET

The Anesthesia Sheet used by the anesthetist during the progress of surgery is a record of the patient's condition throughout the operation. Before the anesthesia is started, the blood pressure, the pulse and the respirations are recorded on the graph on this sheet. The time the anesthesia is started is noted, and continual checks are made by the anesthetist at specific and frequent intervals throughout the time that the patient is on the table. The type of anesthesia used and the route of administration are recorded, as are the drugs administered, the I.V. fluids or blood given, and all other data pertinent to the patient's condition and his physiologic functions. This sheet is part of the patient's permanent record and remains on the chart.

Other monitoring devices may be used by the anesthetist to keep him more accurately informed about the patient's condition, such as continuous electrocardiography. These devices may have their own recording systems and graphs, or their readings may be entered on the anesthesia sheet.

At the end of the operation the circulating nurse signs the entry on the anesthesia sheet for sponge count, stating "sponge count correct."

When the patient is ready to be sent to the recovery room after surgery, all pertinent information about his condition, the number and positions of drains (if any), the retention catheter, chest drainage, etc., is recorded, and the recovery room nurse is informed. This information may be on the back of the record kept by the anesthetist during surgery, or it may be entered separately on a Condition Sheet which accompanies the patient to the recovery room. The important thing is that the information be passed on to the people who will be giving immediate postoperative care to the patient, and that all necessary precautions for his safety and care be taken.

OPERATIVE RECORD

After surgery the surgeon usually dictates his procedure and findings into a recorder. This record then is transcribed by a medical secretary and typed on the operative record sheet for the doctor's review and signature. This then becomes a part of the patient's permanent chart and record.

SPECIAL RECORDS

Circumcision. A special form is used for the parent's consent to a circumcision on an infant. It is a short and abbreviated form because of the nature and the frequency of the surgical procedure. Circumcision should not be done routinely without a consent signed by both parents. If it is done without a signed consent, the hospital and the surgeon may be held liable for damages if a suit is brought against them by the parents.

Death. The report of a death in the operating room goes through prescribed channels on a special form for this purpose. Hospital and operating room policies dictate the information needed on the form and the signatures required (doctor, nurse or others present or involved).

Frozen Section. A Frozen Section Request Form may be used to accompany a biopsy (a small piece of tissue) sent to the laboratory for immediate examination. This is necessary for positive identification of the patient whose tissue is being sent.

Incident Record. An Incident Record (it can be called also an Emergency Report) often is required by hospital policy to be completed whenever an unusual happening occurs to either patients or personnel in or out of the operating room. Such written reports should be made for injuries suffered from accidents, for incorrect sponge counts that evade solution even after x-rays have been taken, for explosions or fire, and for any unique and uncommon occurrences that result in immediate or possible future difficulties. When the information is recorded at the time of the incident, it is more likely to be accurate than if time elapses before the report is made.

REVIEW QUESTIONS:
1. What purpose does a signed consent form serve?
2. Could the preoperative checklist used in your hospital be improved? If so, how?
3. What is the operating room policy in your hospital in relation to the handling of patient charges for surgery? For anesthesia? For special supplies?
4. What type of sponge count sheet is used in your hospital? Does it make the sponge count easier to make and to total?
5. Explain why patient records must be accurate, legible and complete.

Bibliography

Lesnik, M. J., and Anderson, B. E.: Nursing Practice and the Law, ed. 2, pp. 269–270, 284–285, Philadelphia, Lippincott, 1955.
Medicolegal Forms With Legal Analysis, Chicago, Law Department, American Medical Association, 1961.

UNIT 4

Surgical Procedures

CHAPTER 10

THE OPERATION
(Scalpel to Dressings)

IMMEDIATE PREOPERATIVE PREPARATION BY THE SCRUBBED

NURSING ASSISTANT : THE OPERATION BEGINS : HEMOSTASIS :

SPONGE AND TAPE COUNT : SUTURING : DRAINS : CLOSURE

OF A WOUND

IMMEDIATE PREOPERATIVE PREPARATION BY THE SCRUBBED NURSING ASSISTANT

Instruments are arranged conveniently, with those to be used first within easy grasp. A few sutures and ligatures are prepared and placed conveniently. Knife blades after being received (Fig. 82) are placed on knife handles (Fig. 83).

Sponges are counted (p. 187), and those which will be needed early are positioned near the operative site. The suction tip is attached to the tubing, and the set is fixed near the operative area so that it will not slide off the table.

Other preparations peculiar to the specific operation to be performed are made, such as placing clips in a clip holder, connecting pieces of a disassembled instrument and attaching gauze pledgets to an instrument holder.

THE OPERATION BEGINS

The scalpel (knife) for the skin incision is passed to the surgeon or laid on an instrument towel so that the handle is directed to the surgeon's hand. Each assistant is provided with sponges and hemostats. The scalpel and the sponges used on or near the skin are discarded in a specimen basin; they are considered to be contaminated to prevent carrying skin contaminants into the wound. Following the ligation of subcutaneous bleeding vessels, 4 skin towels may be fastened around

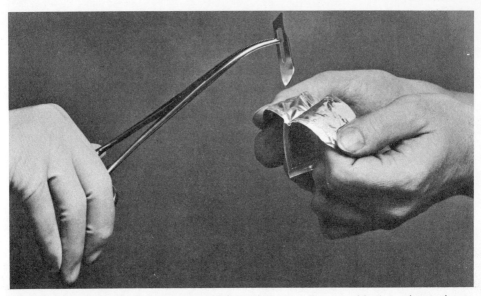

Fig. 82. Circulating nurse peeling back foil wrapper to allow scrubbed nursing assistant to take. (American Safety Razor Company, New York, N.Y.)

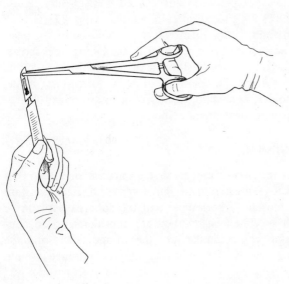

Fig. 83. By grasping the knife blade on the side opposite the cutting edge, a needle holder or a hemostat furnishes a convenient device to position the blade on the handle of the knife. The blade is slipped into the groove on the handle. A click indicates that the blade is in place.

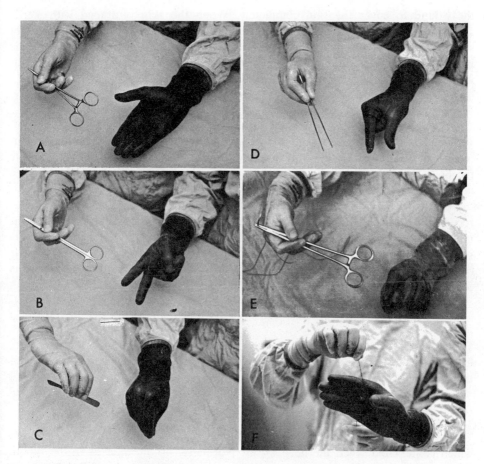

Fig. 84. (A) *Hemostat.* Extend the hand supinated (up). This is the position in which most instruments are received. Even when signals are not being used routinely, this maneuver should be answered with a hemostat unless the surgeon specifically asks for another instrument.

(B) *Scissors.* Extend the index and the middle fingers and adduct and abduct the two fingers in a shearing motion.

(C) *Scalpel.* Hold the hand pronated with the thumb apposed against the distal phalanx of the fingers and flex the wrist.

(D) *Forceps.* Hold the hand pronated (down) and appose the thumb and the index finger. This simulates the position of the hand when holding a forceps.

(E) *Suture.* Extend the hand in a position of bringing the hand from pronation to supination. This simulates holding a needle holder and the motion used in inserting the suture.

(F) *Tie.* Hold the hand elevated with the palm toward the suture nurse. The nurse grasps the tie at each end and sets the midportion in the surgeon's palm. (Nealon, T. F., Jr.: Fundamental Skills in Surgery, pp. 32, 33, Philadelphia, Saunders, 1962)

the wound to cover the skin completely. When the skin is draped with sterile self-adhering plastic drape, it is unnecessary to use skin towels. The advantages of such a waterproof protection over permeable linen drapes are many: (1) plastic is impervious to bacteria and fluids, (2) towel clips are eliminated, and (3) visibility of landmarks is easier (see p. 98).

PASSING INSTRUMENTS

Instruments should be passed in a decisive and positive manner. When an instrument is passed properly, the surgeon knows he has it; his eyes do not have to leave the operative field. When he extends his hand, the instrument should be slapped firmly in his palm in proper position for him to use.

Many surgeons use signals to indicate the type of instrument needed. Such signs speed up the passage of instruments and eliminate unnecessary talking. These signs must be clearly understood and should be reinforced by the technician's understanding of what is taking place at the operative field. Obviously, when there is bleeding, there is need for a hemostat. When a suture needs cutting, the need is for scissors. (Fig. 84)

HEMOSTASIS

The patient's very life may depend on control of bleeding. If a patient is wounded, first aid measures to control bleeding include: application of pressure, elevation of the part, application of cold and inactivity of the area involved.

WAYS OF CONTROLLING BLEEDING

Blood Clotting. Nature has provided human beings with a clotting mechanism which is activated when the need arises. Normally, prothrombin is in the blood. When tissues are injured, thromboplastin is released. The combining of thrombin, thromboplastin and calcium ions produces thrombin within a few minutes. Thrombin combines with the protein fibrinogen to form fibrin, which is the basic structure of a clot.

Hemostat. The surgeon has available many devices and technics for the control of hemorrhage. The most commonly used instrument is the hemostat (hemo = blood; stat = stop). This instrument may vary in size and type of serrations, and it may have a straight or a curved tip; but essentially the purpose is the same: to clamp off a blood vessel. Hemostasis also may be accomplished by torsion (twisting of a blood vessel) or by the use of a ligature.

Ligature. This is a piece of suture material used to tie around a blood vessel that is temporarily clamped by a hemostat. The size and the kind of tying material depend on the size of the blood vessel and the preference of the surgeon.

Heat. Hot packs may be used to control capillary bleeding in extensive operative areas, as in a radical mastectomy.

Oxidized Cellulose (Oxycel,* Surgicel†). This is an absorbable hemostatic agent made of knitted cotton fabric or carded fiber pads. It is placed in or on a bleeding area. It does not adhere to the wound but absorbs blood and swells to become sticky and jellylike (forming coagulum). This coagulum produces hemostasis. Pressure of the cellulose is exerted evenly, since it conforms to the contour of the wound.

Gelatin Sponge, Powder or Film. This is made from specially cured and sterilized gelatin. The sponge or foam hastens clot formation, stops bleeding and promotes tissue repair. In pack form it can be used to fill dead space from which sizable amounts of tissue have been removed. Gelatin powder is taken by mouth to aid in hemostasis in gastroduodenal bleeding. Gelatin film, which is a thin transparent sheet, is used in replacing injured dura (brain cover) or pleura (lung covering). Such a film can be cut into the required size and remains intact for about 90 days before it gradually is replaced by connective tissue.

Thrombin. This is a powder made from beef blood. It can be sprinkled directly on an oozing surface or applied topically in solution form. Thrombin controls capillary bleeding and hastens blood coagulation.

Bone wax is used to seal bleeders from bone. It is made essentially from beeswax.

Electrosurgery. This is the process of using high-frequency electrical energy for controlled cutting, dehydration or destruction of tissue.

Surgical Diathermy. By means of a needle or a knifelike tip attached to a handle and connected to an electric machine by a cord, the surgeon is able to sear tissue as a means of controlling bleeding. The electric current heats the metal tip or electrode by means of high-frequency current. This passes through the patient's body between two electrodes: (1) the electrode or operative tip used by the surgeon and described above, and (2) the large stainless steel plate that is placed under the patient in direct contact with the skin. This must be lubricated to provide close contact with the skin, and it is connected by means of a cord to the machine. (Fig. 86)

By turning a handle on the diathermy machine, the surgeon can do one of three things: (1) electrocoagulation, i.e., the searing of tissue to control bleeding, (2) cutting, or (3) desiccation, making the tissue very dry.

Electrode tip attachments vary in size and style. The more common kinds are needles, knives, loops and coagulating balls.

Electrocautery (Downes cautery). This is a device that heats a wire electrode to red heat for the purpose of burning tissue areas. A smaller unit than the surgical diathermy apparatus, the electrocautery often is used to cut and cauterize the appendix, to cut across the stomach and the intestine, and to open a colostomy. The cautery consists of a transformer, encased in a wooden box, which heats the cautery tip or the knife. A numbered dial is used to indicate heat intensity. Tips or knives

---

* Parke, Davis Co.   † Johnson and Johnson.

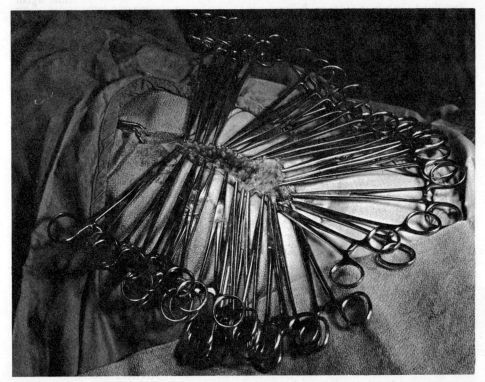

Fig. 85. Hemostasis is accomplished by clamping vessels with sharply pointed small hemostats, then removing the hemostats as the vessels are tied with fine cotton ligatures (or other suitable material). It is preferable to conserve the patient's own blood with the application of many hemostats rather than to replace lost blood by transfusion. (Harkins, H. N., *et al.*: Surgery, Principles and Practice, ed. 2, p. 223, Philadelphia, Lippincott, 1961) (*Continued on facing page*)

SAFETY PRECAUTIONS FOR DIATHERMY AND CAUTERY

Check that proper attachments of all cords and metal plates are made.

Follow safety regulations when explosive anesthetic agents may be present.

Start at lowest current and work up to desired intensity required by the surgeon to do the task. Increase current only at surgeon's request.

Keep flammable liquids, such as alcohol and ether, well away from these units.

Be familiar with operating instruction booklet which accompanies the unit.

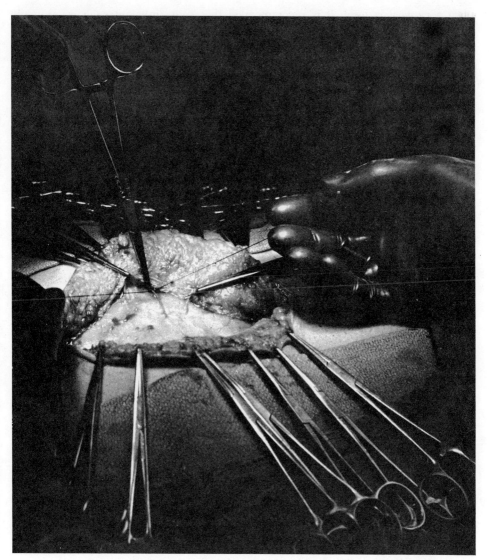

Fig. 85 (*Cont.*)

are interchangeable, although some handles have fixed knives.

Precautions must be observed when the cautery is used to prevent explosion and injury to the apparatus itself. The dial is turned as high as necessary to do the task; but if it is turned too high, the tip or the blade can melt and injure the patient. Alcohol and alcohol sponges are kept away from the cautery, because alcohol ignites readily. Wet saline sponges are placed around the area where the cautery is to be used. Since the conscious patient may be upset by the odor of burned tissue when a cautery is used, it is recommended that some inhalant such as aromatic spirits of ammonia on a sponge be available for him to smell. (Fig. 87).

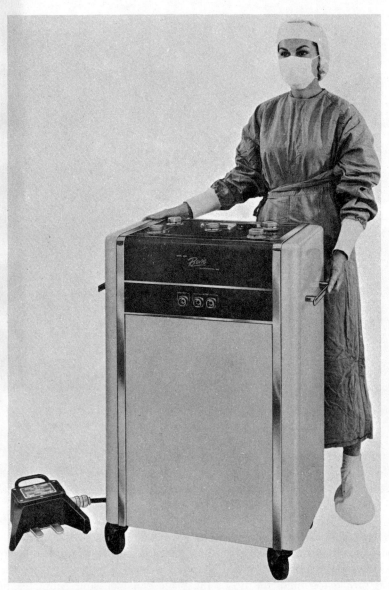

Fig. 86. Bovie electrosurgical unit. Note the safety connection between the foot pedal and the machine. (Ritter Equipment Company, a Division of Ritter Company, Inc., Rochester, N.Y.) (*Continued on facing page*)

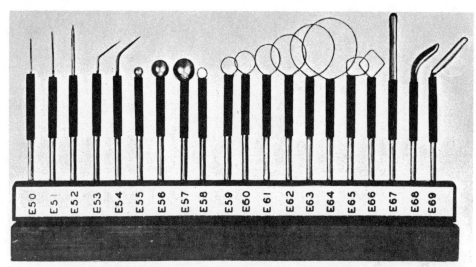

Fig. 86 (*Cont.*). Surgical diathermy electrodes. From left to right are needle, ball, loop and knife electrodes. (Hall, E. D.: Surgical Instrument Guide for Nurses, Brooklyn, N.Y., Weck, 1954)

Other Forms of Hemostasis. *Styptic.* This is a chemical which causes constriction or contraction of blood vessels (an astringent) and coagulates blood albumin. An example of a styptic is epinephrine, which is used in direct application to mucous membranes (nasal surgery) and in local anesthetics.

Clips. Small silver clips bent in the shape of V are used by neurosurgeons in a special clip holder to clamp blood vessels in brain surgery.

Vitamin K. This is administered preoperatively and postoperatively to aid in blood coagulation.

SPONGE AND TAPE COUNT

An accounting of all sponges and tapes is done to prevent the loss of a sponge in a patient. Such an oversight can cause serious harm to the patient, because the sponge is a foreign object to which the body reacts in a defensive manner. Expensive legal suits have resulted from such carelessness.

Although most hospitals have elaborate methods of counting and recording sponges for certain operative procedures, the same concern and diligent precautions are taken to prevent leaving anything in a wound, such as an instrument, a needle or a cotton pledget. Packs, drains and catheters that are to remain in a wound must be fastened to dressings and properly identified.

Counted sponges and tapes are used if a body cavity is entered, or if the operating field is large or deep or has pockets in which a sponge could be overlooked. In the following operations counted sponges are likely to be used:

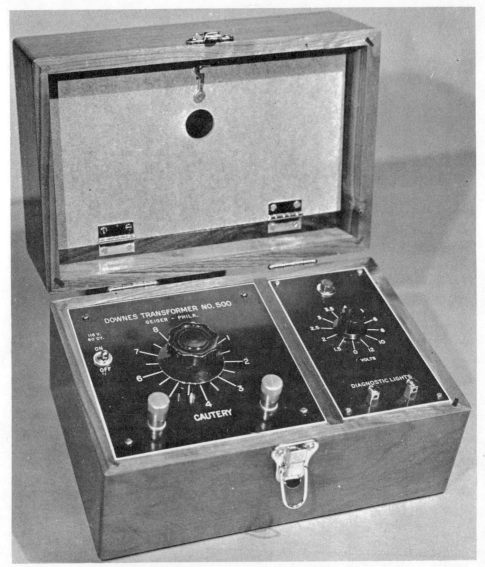

Fig. 87 (A). Downes cautery transformer.

Laparotomy, including herniorrhaphy
Radical mastectomy
Thoracic operations
Kidney, ureter and bladder surgery
Substernal thyroidectomy

Abdominal and vaginal hysterectomy
Hip or femur operations
Spinal surgery (occasionally)

Types of Sponges

Counted sponges and tapes are made differently from uncounted sponges. To facilitate counting,

1. Uncounted gauze sponges are removed from the operating field.

2. Metal rings (1½" in diameter) are looped through double-twilled tape fastened to a corner of a sponge. These rings dangle from the wound edge while the attached sponges are in the wound.

3. When gauze sponges are used in a deep cavity, they usually are placed on a sponge forceps and handed on an exchange basis, only one at a time.

4. Sponges and tapes with x-ray-detectable thread can be purchased. If special sponges are made at the hospital, radiopaque thread should be stitched into the sponge.

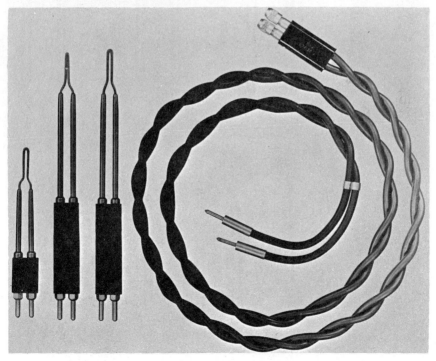

Fig. 87 (B). Downes cautery cable and cautery knives with attached handles.

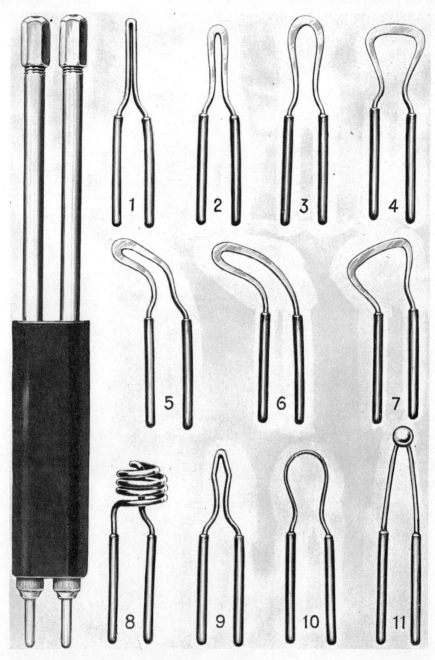

Fig. 87 (C). Downes cautery tips. (Geiger Instrument Co., Inc., Philadelphia)

Counting and Recording

A common and effective procedure is for sponges and tapes to be counted at 3 or 4 different times for one operation. Two persons count sponges in an audible voice as each sponge is separated in the counting process. Sponges are counted:

1. By the persons who wrap them prior to sterilization. (This may be a machine count done by the company who manufactures precounted radiopaque sponges.)

2. By the circulating and scrub nurse immediately before the operation starts and as each additional package is needed. The circulating nurse records the count.

3. When the closure of the wound is begun. This usually is done by the surgeon, or his first assistant, and the circulating and scrub nurse.

4. After the peritoneum has been closed or if a discrepancy in the count is noted.

Management of Sponges During the Operation

As counted sponges and tapes are used, they can be discarded conveniently in a large kidney basin placed near the operative field. Such a receptacle discourages the practice of tossing soiled sponges on the floor. The scrub nurse empties the kidney basin into a kick bucket placed conveniently near her and in her line of vision.

A small amount of water in the bottom of the bucket will reduce the hazard of static electricity created by the large polyethylene bag that is placed in the bucket and draped over the outside. The circulating nurse is able to separate and drape each sponge over the edge of the bucket until 10 are collected. At a convenient time she and the scrub nurse count the sponges as they are deposited in a plastic or waterproof bag, which is tied and placed on a table to await the final count. To avoid the positive transmission of hepatitis, *soiled sponges never are touched with bare hands. The circulator uses sponge forceps or gloved hands.*

Sponge racks are undesirable in an operating room, because they are unsightly, may contribute to the number of airborne organisms and are difficult to clean.

At the end of the operation or after the peritoneum is closed, a final sponge count is taken. If it is correct, the circulating nurse reports to the surgeon and signs the operative record to indicate the correct count.

If the count is incorrect, a thorough search is made immediately for the missing sponges. Favorite hiding places are the wound, the folds of drapes, under towels or pans, and occasionally with a specimen that has been sent to the pathology laboratory. A recounting of all sponges in bags may be necesary, which is the reason that they are not to be removed from the room. Hospital policy should make mandatory the taking of an x-ray picture when the sponge count is incorrect. An incident report and a notation on the operative record also must be made.

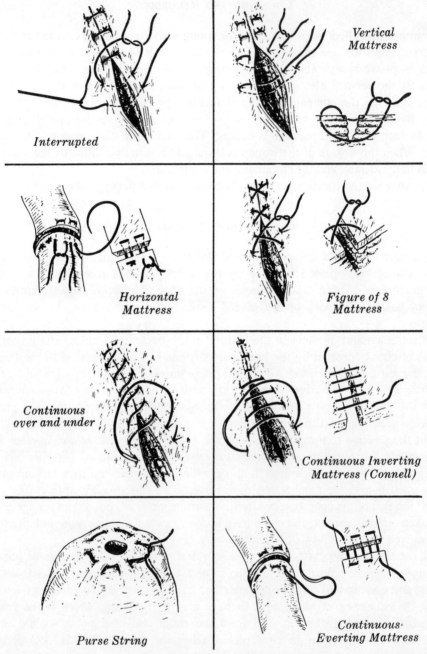

Interrupted

Vertical Mattress

Horizontal Mattress

Figure of 8 Mattress

Continuous over and under

Continuous Inverting Mattress (Connell)

Purse String

Continuous Everting Mattress

Fig. 88. Types of surgical stitching. (Davis & Geck Suture Manual, p. 44, Danbury, Conn., American Cyanamid Company, 1963)

SUTURING

TYPES OF STITCHES

Just as a housewife uses a variety of stitches—basting, hemstitch and backstitch—
to create a new garment, so does a surgeon use different kinds of stitches to close a
wound. The type of stitch used depends on the surgeon's preference and the nature
of the tissue to be approximated (brought together). These conditions influence
not only the type of suture to be used but also the length of the suture to be
prepared. For instance, in an *interrupted suture,* which sometimes is used on the
skin, a stitch is taken, then tied and cut. A short length of suture is required for
this type of stitch. For a *continuous suture,* which generally is used to close the
peritoneal layer, the surgeon begins to sew at one point, ties and continues to suture
until the end of the incision has been reached. This technic is like the hemming
of a skirt. Obviously, a long length of suture material is required. A *purse-string
suture,* which sometimes is used on the base of the appendix, is a continuous stitch
formed in a circle that ends in a drawstring; it is used when it is desirable to invert
cut edges of tissue. A medium length suture is required for this technic.

THREADING AN EYED NEEDLE

(See also Chap. 5, p. 73.) A suture is threaded in such a way that one strand is
longer than the other; the short end should be about 3 inches. It is disturbing to the
surgeon to have the suture pull out or fall out of the needle before he has a chance
to use it. Two ways of helping to prevent this are: (1) to thread the curved needle
from the inner curve to the outer curve, and (2) to give a twist to the threaded
suture close to the eye of the needle.

ACCOUNTING FOR NEEDLES

While the surgeon is using one suture, the scrubbed assistant should be threading
the next one. As one becomes familiar with the operation and the surgeon's preferences, the kind of needle, the size and the type of suture material are readily
learned. A system of keeping track of needles needs to be followed, so that all
needles are accounted for, and none is lost. Likewise, it is important that the
needle be intact; if a needle should break, all parts must be retrieved. Remember
that although swaged needles are threaded commercially, they must be intact and
accounted for when they are returned by the surgeon.

POSITIONING THE NEEDLE AND PASSING A SUTURE

Straight needles are threaded so that the short end is no longer than 3 inches. The
eyed and atraumatic straight needles are handed directly to the surgeon and not

fixed on a needle holder. The passer holds the needle near the middle with the point visible and the threaded end exposed for the surgeon to grasp.

A suture with a curved needle is handed to the surgeon so that it is ready to have the point directed to the tissue to be stitched. The long end of the suture usually is passed to the first assistant, and the surgeon is provided with a pair of forceps. Scissors are made available to the surgeon's assistant. Whether the surgeon is on the same side of the operating table as the scrubbed assistant or on the opposite side will determine the way of passing both instruments and sutures: they should be ready for him to use immediately.

DRAINS

Wounds are drained to remove excess fluid and air. Drainage in some instances, like that from the chest, the gallbladder, the common bile duct or the bladder, passes directly through the tube. In other instances, like that from the peritoneal cavity, drainage of accumulated pus or blood passes primarily along the outside surface of the drain.

The most common type of drainage tube is a thin-walled rubber tube (Penrose) which may or may not contain a gauze wick. Such a tube should have sufficient lumen to carry secretions and should be of adequate thickness to prevent collapse. The drain is inserted in the area where oozing is expected. Because in most areas of the body pressure is greater than atmospheric pressure, secretions tend to flow outward (the exception is the thoracic cavity, in which a lower than atmospheric pressure exists). In a cholecystectomy, gauze-filled Penrose drains are used commonly in the space formerly occupied by the gallbladder. It is possible to pull this drain out gradually at postoperative dressing time and leave a shortened segment in the wound.

The *sump drain* is used in wounds in which there may be excessive or irritating drainage from a large cavity or abscess. It varies as to type. One kind is a single rubber tube with multiple perforations; the other consists of two perforated tubes, one within the other. A sump drain usually is attached to a continuous suction unit.

CLOSURE OF A WOUND

PRIMARY SUTURE LINE

For healing by *first intention,* the surgeon sutures each layer of tissue separately, thereby approximating the complete wound margin. This technic results in what is called the *primary suture line.* (Fig. 89)

SECONDARY SUTURE LINE

For some patients the surgeon may request a *secondary suture line.* This is necessary when the surgeon seeks to relieve strain on the primary suture line, to obliterate dead space, or to prevent the accumulation of blood and serum in the

Fig. 89. Primary suture line. Each layer
is sutured separately. (Davis &
Geck Suture Manual, p. 45, Danbury, Conn., American Cyanamid Company, 1963)

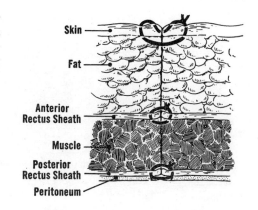

wound. Sutures used for this purpose are called stay sutures, tension sutures or
through-and-through sutures. To prevent the tension suture from cutting into the
skin, a piece of rubber or plastic tubing often called a "boot" or "bumper" may be
threaded through the exposed suture before it is tied.

SUTURELESS SKIN CLOSURE

For many years medical researchers have looked for ways to avoid the necessity
of puncturing the skin with suture needles, since skin cannot be sterilized despite
careful and meticulous cleaning procedures. Therefore, other methods of securing
wound margins were sought. Now available is a specially designed surgical adhesive
tape which is made into sterile strips, is physiologically inert, permits ventilation
of the skin, and provides secure bonding on the wound, but release is easy when
this is required. An ever-increasing number of surgeons are using this type of skin
closure for patients.

REVIEW QUESTIONS:
 1. How does blood clotting take place?
 2. Describe how oxidized cellulose produces hemostasis.
 3. Where does bone wax come from? For what is it used?
 4. Why are two electrodes necessary in surgical diathermy?
 5. What is the difference between electrocoagulation and desiccation?
 6. What safety precautions should be practiced when using diathermy and cautery?
 7. Evaluate the sponge count procedure in your hospital. Could it be im-
    proved?
 8. Why are soiled sponges never touched with bare hands?
 9. Differentiate between a purse-string suture and a continuous suture.
10. What is a sump drain?
11. What is the difference between a primary suture line and a secondary suture
    line?
12. What are the advantages of sutureless wound closure?

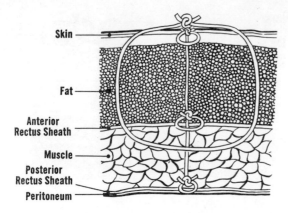

Skin

Fat

Anterior
Rectus Sheath

Muscle

Posterior
Rectus Sheath

Peritoneum

Fig. 90. Secondary suture line. A line of sutures passing through several layers of tissue and placed on each side of the primary suture line. (Davis & Geck Suture Manual, p. 47, Danbury, Conn., American Cyanamid Company, 1963)

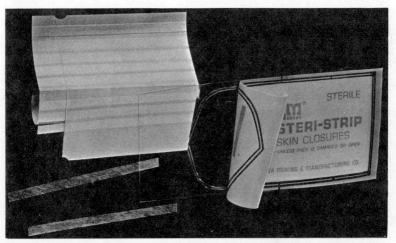

Fig. 91. Steri-strips. (Minnesota Mining and Manufacturing Company, St. Paul, Minn.)

Bibliography

Alexander, E. L.: Care of the Patient in Surgery (including techniques), ed. 3, St. Louis, Mosby, 1958.

Davis and Geck Suture Manual, Danbury, Conn., American Cyanamid Company, 1963.

Ethicon Manual of Operative Procedure and Surgical Knots, Somerville, N.J., Ethicon, Inc., 1961.

Ginsberg, F.: Modern sponge precautions can prevent operating room grief, Mod. Hosp. 101:122, July 1963; 101:129, August 1963.

Hall, E. D.: Surgical Instrument Guide for Nurses, Brooklyn, N.Y., Weck, 1954.

Rockwell, V. T.: Sponge counts and blood loss determinations, A.O.R.N.J. 1:52–60, November–December, 1963.

CHAPTER 11

SOME COMMON SURGICAL CONDITIONS AND OPERATIVE PROCEDURES

INTRODUCTION : TONSILLECTOMY AND ADENOIDECTOMY :

SURGERY OF THE BREAST : APPENDECTOMY : SURGERY OF THE

BILIARY SYSTEM : GASTRECTOMY : HEMORRHOIDS AND OTHER

RECTAL PROBLEMS : D. AND C. OPERATION : CYSTOSCOPY : VEIN

LIGATION AND STRIPPING : ORTHOPEDIC SURGERY

INTRODUCTION

This chapter is concerned with a description of a number of operative procedures. They are the kind of operations that may be found on almost any operating room schedule. The intent of the authors is to convey an over-all understanding of basic operative procedures that may facilitate the later learning of the specific details of instrumentation, sutures, draping, etc., as they apply to individual patients in particular hospitals.

TONSILLECTOMY AND ADENOIDECTOMY
(T. and A. Surgery)

A tonsillectomy and adenoidectomy is a surgical procedure done to remove the tonsils and the adenoids. The tonsils are two masses of glandlike tissue that are embedded in each side of the throat (the pharynx just behind and above the level of the tongue). Normally, they measure about 1½ inches long by ¾ of an inch

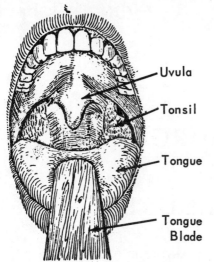

Uvula

Tonsil

Tongue

Tongue
Blade

Fig. 92. Diagrammatic view of tonsils. (Brunner, L. S., et al.: Medical-Surgical Nursing, p. 383, Philadelphia, Lippincott, 1964)

wide and are barely visible on throat examination. The adenoids usually are one fused clump of glandlike tissue about half the size of the tonsils. The adenoids lie on the back of the throat above the level of the soft palate and cannot be seen during routine throat examinations. (Figs. 92, 93)

Tonsil and adenoid tissue is thought to serve as a barrier to or strainer of microorganisms, localizing infection and giving the body some immunity to organisms that enter the body through the nose and the mouth. When these tissues become inflamed, they enlarge and sometimes drain, causing persistent sore throat, high fever, and often swollen neck glands. In some instances enlarged and infected adenoids, because of the proximity of the eustachian tubes, cause loss of hearing and ear infections, and they may interfere with normal respiration, with the result that patients become "mouth breathers." Until recently, physicians recommended T. and A. surgery for all children when they reached the 3- to 5-age group. Current more conservative professional judgment advises that surgery be done only when there is indication of disease or complications.

Normally, after a child reaches the age of 10, tonsil and adenoid tissue tends to shrink. By the time that the child reaches maturity, adenoid tissue in particular reduces to a size that rarely causes difficulties. For this reason a tonsillectomy performed on an adult does not include an adenoidectomy.

A T. and A. performed on a child usually is done under general anesthesia. The anesthetized child generally is placed flat on his back, with his head lower than his feet. This position prevents blood from being aspirated (taken into lungs or stomach). A tonsillectomy performed on an adult usually is done under local anesthesia with the patient in a sitting position, since the adult can keep the operative field clear by expectoration at appropriate moments.

Fig. 93. Diagrammatic cross section drawing to show the parts of the upper respiratory tract and their relation to each other. (Brunner, L. S., *et al.:* Medical-Surgical Nursing, p. 378, Philadelphia, Lippincott, 1964)

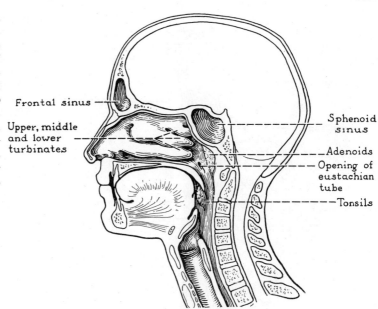

Frontal sinus

Upper, middle and lower turbinates

Sphenoid sinus

Adenoids

Opening of eustachian tube

Tonsils

If the patient is under general anesthesia, the mouth retractor is placed carefully, the ether hook is attached, and the surgeon retracts tissue to visualize his incisional site. Using a tonsil knife, he incises the mucous membrane and frees the tonsil through blunt dissection until it is attached only at its base. The tissues involved are highly vascular (rich in blood supply), and the control of bleeding is of real concern to the surgeon. Throat suctioning is very important because it removes blood that collects at the base of the mouth. The suction tip must be secured tightly to the instrument, and frequent flushing in water is necessary to keep the tubing clear. Grasping the tonsil securely, the surgeon snips the tissue off at its base with a snare or a cutting instrument. The remaining hole (fossa) is carefully inspected for tonsil tabs, and bleeding vessels are clamped. Finally, a tonsil sponge with a securely tied string is introduced into the fossa for pressure to stop the bleeding of small vessels. The string is permitted to drape the face while the second tonsil is removed in a similar manner. When both tonsils have been removed, the surgeon introduces a cutting instrument, called an adenotome, through the mouth behind the uvula into the adenoid area and removes the adenoid tissue. An adenoid curette is used to determine the presence of remaining tabs of tissue, and after finger palpation (feeling) the surgeon inserts a long-stringed adenoid sponge until hemostasis has been accomplished. When all of the stringed-sponges have been removed, the area is carefully inspected to insure a dry field. If a cut vessel begins to bleed, it is clamped and may be tied with a piece of fine plain surgical gut.

The patient is placed in a crib or on a stretcher with his head turned to one side

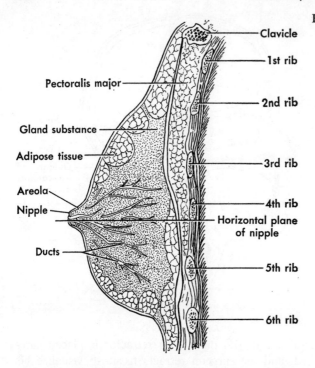

Fig. 94. Right breast in sagittal section, inner surface of outer segment, (Kimber, D. C., *et al.:* Anatomy and Physiology, ed. 14, p. 696, Fig. 394, New York, Macmillan, 1961)

during the postanesthetic period. If bleeding or vomiting occurs, the patient in this position is cared for readily. He is watched carefully through the recovery period to be certain that blood and vomitus are not aspirated into the lungs.

SURGERY OF THE FEMALE BREAST

The breast is a glandular organ which includes a network of ducts that carry milk to the nipple. Throughout the breast there is a rich supply of blood and lymphatic fluid (Fig. 94). By a complicated process milk results from the transforming of amino acids and glucose into proteins and lactose. Hormones secreted by the ovary affect lactation. For example, estrogen is an ovarian hormone that suppresses the formation of milk, whereas progesterone stimulates lactation.

The function of the female breast is to provide nourishment to the newborn and young infant. In most women in our society, this function is limited to a few weeks or months if the mother nurses at all. Authorities agree that an organ which is not used fully is more likely to become diseased than an active organ. Further problems may be caused by the necessity of the normal breast to adjust to changes in structure and function as each woman passes through various cycles. These progress from adolescence through the menstrual cycles to pregnancy, lactation and the menopause. Another factor which accounts for breast difficulties is the un-protected position of the breast, which exposes it to injury.

DISORDERS OF THE BREAST

Fissure or a "crack" in the nipple can occur during the time that a mother nurses her baby. The sucking action of the baby causes further irritation, pain and bleed-ing, which prevents healing. By following good hygienic principles, such as cleansing and drying the nipple before and after nursing, this problem will be prevented.

Mastitis and Abscess. Inflammation of the breast (mastitis) and subsequent abscess formation can occur when infection is present. Treatment consists of keep-ing the area clean, using antibiotics, and, if need be, incision and drainage.

Cysts. Another difficulty may be the occurrence of cysts (abnormal collection of fluid within a definite sac or wall). These appear as firm, smooth round masses and may be tender on palpation. Treatment is usually *aspiration* (withdrawal of fluid using a syringe and a needle). When cysts are combined with inflammation, a condition of *cystic mastitis* is produced. The cysts feel like tiny lead shots. This should be observed carefully for a time by the physician.

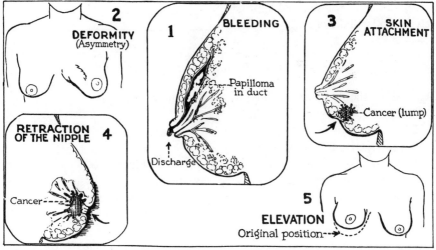

Fig. 95. Signs of cancer of the breast. (1) Bleeding from the nipple arising from a papilloma in the duct. This may be a benign lesion at first, but it is defi-nitely considered to be a premalignant lesion. (2) Deformity or asymmetry of the breast. (3) Skin attachment at the site of a malignant mass. (4) Re-traction of the nipple when cancer appears at the center of the breast. (5) Elevation of the breast involved due to contraction and shortening of the fibrous tissue trabeculations brought about by the malignant tumor. (American Cancer Society, New York)

Tumor problems of the breast (a tumor is an abnormal growth of tissue) fall into two categories: (1) Benign (nonmalignant) and (2) malignant.

A *benign tumor* is a type which grows slowly and encloses itself in a capsule. It exerts pressure on the surrounding area but does not invade the nearby tissues. When this tumor is removed, it does not grow back.

A *malignant tumor* is also called *cancer* or a *neoplasm*. Such a growth invades the tissues, much like an octopus reaching out with tentacles. Unlike the benign tumor, the malignant growth is not surrounded by a capsule. A malignant tumor invades blood vessels and lymphatic channels. Tumor cells often are broken off and carried by these vessels or channels to other parts of the body, where they can lodge and set up a new growth. Such spreading of a cancer is called *metastasis*.

Breast cancer strikes about 1 in every 18 women in this country. It is estimated that 65,000 American women in 1966 will acquire this condition, and approximately 27,000 will die of it.

> SEVEN CARDINAL SIGNS
> OF CANCER
>
> 1. A sore which does not heal within 2 weeks.
> 2. A lump or mass in the breast or elsewhere in the body.
> 3. Unusual bleeding or discharge from any body opening (orifice).
> 4. Changes in the shape, the size or the appearance of a wart or a mole.
> 5. Continuing indigestion or difficulty in swallowing.
> 6. Hoarseness or cough that does not clear within 2 weeks.
> 7. Any changes in normal bowel habits.

DETECTION OF PROBLEMS OF THE BREAST

Signs which should be investigated by a physician are:
1. A lump.
2. Ulceration.
3. An enlarged gland in the armpit.
4. The above signs plus any of the signs shown in Figure 96.

Any of the foregoing signs should be investigated by a physician so that an accurate and early diagnosis can be made. Although pain as a symptom usually is not a sign of early cancer, it also should be investigated, because it may be related to some other condition.

Several diagnostic procedures are available to the physician. *Inspection* and *palpation* of the breast are the most common and consist of the physician's gently examining breast tissue with the palm of his hand in an attempt to detect a lump. *Mammography* or x-ray of the breast is done in some clinics; this is a more expensive diagnostic aid, but physicians who favor it claim that cancer can be detected much earlier this way. *Biopsy* is the removal of a piece of tissue for microscopic examination. Usually this procedure is done in an operating room under general anesthesia.

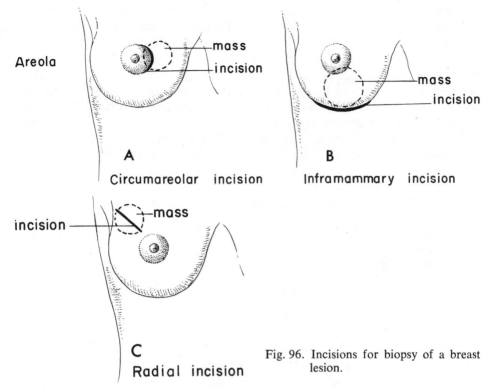

Areola

A
Circumareolar incision

B
Inframammary incision

C
Radial incision

Fig. 96. Incisions for biopsy of a breast lesion.

On confirmation of the diagnosis of cancer by the laboratory report, the surgical team prepares for and performs a mastectomy.

OPERATIVE PROCEDURES FOR BIOPSY AND RADICAL MASTECTOMY

Biopsy. If the lesion is beneath or near the areola, the skin incision is made in a curved fashion so that on healing the scar is not obvious (Fig. 97A). If the mass is deep and near the lower surface, an inframammary incision is used (Fig. 97B). Other incisions in the breast usually are reached by a radial incision (Fig. 97C). This opening radiates out from the nipple.

The tumor specimen is sent immediately to the laboratory for a *frozen section* examination. In this procedure the tissue is frozen rapidly, usually with a jet spray of CO_2; then very thin slices containing a good cross section of cells is placed on a glass slide and tinted with a dye to make observation under the microscope more vivid. Meanwhile, the incision site is closed with sutures. If the laboratory report indicates that the tissue is benign, the patient is returned to her room. However, if cancer cells are detected, the operating team changes gown and gloves, the patient is redraped, and the major set-up for mastectomy is moved into place. Further laboratory studies of the specimen are pursued later.

Mastectomy. The incision is usually an elliptical one, as illustrated in Figure 97. However, it often is tailored to the needs of the individual patient. When dissection or removal of the axillary lymph nodes is done, the incision may be directed toward the axilla. The surgeon cuts under the skin area, as shown in the shaded portion of Figure 97, to free enough skin and underlying fat so that the edges may be brought together more easily after breast removal. Rake retractors are used to expose the area of dissection. In some clinics sponges are counted. Large bands of muscles, the pectoralis major and the pectoralis minor, are freed and cut before the surgeon dissects the axillary tissue. All bleeding points are clamped and ligated; the wound is cleaned. The skin edges are brought together and sutured. If drainage is desired, a stab wound is made in the axillary region and a soft rubber tube or Penrose drain is inserted. Some surgeons include retention sutures. In the event that the skin edges do not approximate (come together), it may be necessary to apply a skin graft.

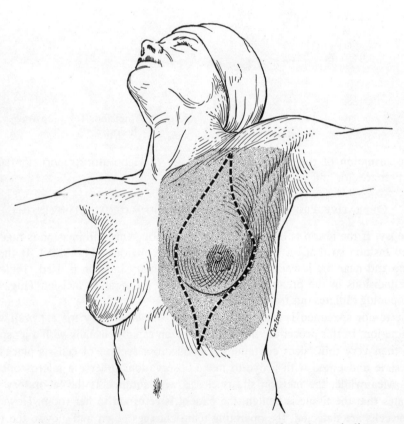

Fig. 97. Usual incision for a radical mastectomy. Shaded area indicates undercutting. (Garside, E., and Mella, L.: Radical mastectomy, Surg. Clin. N. Am. 41:180, Fig. 1, February 1961)

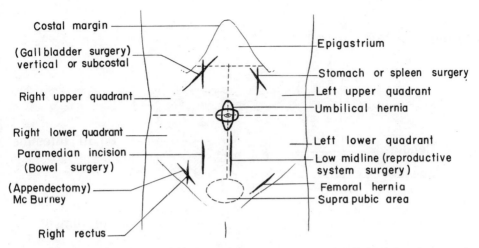

Costal margin

(Gall bladder surgery)
vertical or subcostal

Right upper quadrant

Right lower quadrant

Paramedian incision
(Bowel surgery)

(Appendectomy)
Mc Burney

Right rectus

Epigastrium

Stomach or spleen surgery

Left upper quadrant

Umbilical hernia

Left lower quadrant

Low midline (reproductive
system surgery)

Femoral hernia

Supra pubic area

Fig. 98. Typical abdominal incisional sites. The abdomen can be divided into four quadrants. Some of the more common incisions are indicated.

Usually, this is done by taking skin from the anterior thigh. Such a graft may be done at the time of mastectomy or at a later date. Dressings are applied; fluffed gauzes may be placed in the axilla and around the drain to aid in compression. A binder then may be applied to compress the affected arm to the chest. Such pressure aids in the prevention of postoperative swelling of the operative site and the arm.

APPENDECTOMY

The removal of the appendix is the most common of all operations requiring abdominal surgery. In addition, the operation often is performed in conjunction with other operations requiring abdominal surgery, i.e., cholecystectomy (removal of gallbladder), oophorectomy (removal of ovary).

The appendix, an organ with no known function, is located at the base of the cecum (first part of large intestine). It is a small, wormlike blind sac that normally is about the width of a lead pencil and measures between 1½ and 7 inches in length. The lumen fills with fecal material, and it frequently becomes inflamed, infected or gangrenous (when the blood supply has been impaired). With any change from the normal, the appendix may enlarge to 8 to 10 times its usual size and cause symptoms that resemble disease in almost any other abdominal organ. In its usual position it projects down from the cecum, but the appendix is highly mobile and may be found in any one of a number of positions within the abdominal cavity.

Acute appendicitis occurs in both sexes and at any age, although it is most common in young adults in their 20's to 40's. The symptoms, which vary widely, generally include abdominal pain and cramps, nausea and vomiting, and elevated

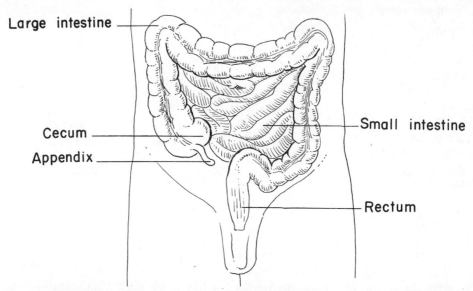

Fig. 99. Diagrammatic drawing showing the relation of the appendix to the large and the small intestines.

temperature. A blood count usually shows a significant increase in the white blood cell count (which indicates inflammation or infection).

When symptoms appear, surgery generally is immediate. Waiting could entail the onset of peritonitis (inflammation of the peritoneal layer), which might seriously threaten the patient's life.

An appendectomy can be the simplest of all the major operations, or it can be very difficult, depending on the position of the organ and the degree of involvement with other tissues. The procedure takes anywhere from 20 minutes to 2 hours, depending on the complications. Since the procedure demands that the abdominal cavity be entered, nursing service personnel assisting the surgeon make an accurate listing of all the sponges to be used.

An appendectomy is performed with the patient in supine position (flat on his back), usually under general anesthesia. In some hospitals spinal anesthesia is preferred. After careful preparation of the skin and application of sterile drapes, the surgeon makes either a McBurney incision (an oblique muscle-splitting incision 2 to 4 inches long in the right lower quadrant) or a longitudinal incision (see Fig. 92). Following careful layer-by-layer dissection while maintaining hemostasis, the surgeon explores, identifies and delivers the appendix into the wound. The mesoappendix (the fatty tissue that anchors the appendix to the intestine) is freed, the important arteries are clamped and ligated, and the appendix generally is double-clamped at its base; then it is tied off, cut and removed. The surrounding tissues are protected with a moist sponge to avoid any contact with chemicals. The remaining stump often is cauterized with an applicator moistened in carbolic acid and then neutralized with alcohol. Some surgeons use a fine purse-string suture to invert the stump. When complications of pus and peritonitis are present, the surgeon inserts one or two Penrose (thin rubber tissue) drains within the abdominal cavity to continue drainage. As soon as the wound closure begins, nursing personnel recount all sponges to be certain that none has been left within the cavity. After the final dressing is applied, the patient is moved to the recovery room for further careful observation. In· uncomplicated cases the patient usually is ambulatory (walking about) the day after surgery.

SURGERY OF THE BILIARY SYSTEM

THE BILIARY SYSTEM

The biliary system is made up primarily of the *liver* and the *gallbladder* as well as the following ducts (tubes):
1. *Hepatic duct,* coming from the liver.
2. *Cystic duct,* coming from the gallbladder.
3. *Pancreatic duct,* coming from the pancreas.

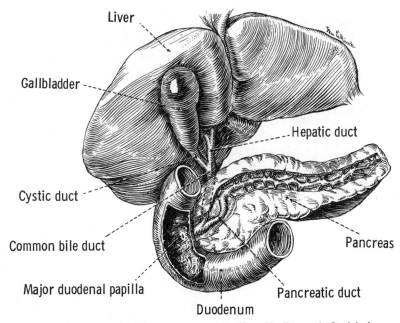

Fig. 100. The normal biliary system. (Chaffee, E. E., and Greisheimer, E. M.: Basic Physiology and Anatomy, p. 487, Philadelphia, Lippincott, 1964)

These ducts in turn unite to form the *common bile duct,* which eventually enters the small intestine. (The biliary system often is referred to as the biliary tree because of its branched shape.)

The *liver* is the largest gland in the body, very rich in blood supply; in the average adult it weighs about 3 pounds. Resembling beef liver in structure and texture, the human liver is located in the upper part of the abdomen on the right side, just under the diaphragm and above the duodenum and the lower end of the stomach. The most important function of the liver is to produce *bile,* a digestive juice. The liver also changes glucose (simple sugar) to glycogen and stores it until it is needed by the body. It stores protein, iron, copper and vitamins; it plays an important part in destroying bacteria and worn-out blood cells; it reduces the toxoid effects of poisons and medicines; it assists in the production of antibodies for defense against disease. These functions and many others make the liver an organ that is essential to life; therefore it cannot be removed completely.

The production of bile begins with bile pigments (the chief of which is bilirubin) carried to the liver by the blood. Within the small lobules (manufacturing plants) which make up the liver, the secreted bile contains about 90 per cent water, bile pigments, cholesterol, bile salts and other chemicals. Bile is drained by many small ducts which eventually empty into the right and the left bile ducts. These join to become the *hepatic duct.* Bile is needed by the body to emulsify (break up) fat particles so that other chemicals of the digestive process can act more quickly and easily on food.

The *gallbladder* is a small pear-shaped sac lodged in a hollow on the under side of the liver. It is connected to the biliary tree by means of the cystic duct, which normally has the diameter of an ordinary lead pencil. The main function of the gallbladder is the storage and the concentration of bile when it is not needed for digestion.

DISORDERS OF THE BILIARY SYSTEM

This part of the body is subject to many kinds of disorders. *Cirrhosis of the liver* is a condition that results from changes due to destruction and scar tissue formation of some of the liver lobules. *Jaundice* (icterus) occurs in diseases of the liver or the biliary apparatus when bile enters the blood stream instead of being eliminated into the intestine. A common condition that may become a surgical problem is the formation of *gallstones,* which may obstruct the cystic and/or common bile ducts (cholelithiasis).

As far back as the early days of the Talmud, references can be found to gallbladder disease and gallstones. A reasonable assumption is that as man's diet became rich in a variety of foods, as he grew heavier and indulged in less physical exercise, his gallbladder became less efficient and therefore prone to the formation of gallstones. In our society the overeating of heavy, rich foods can cause disorders of this organ. Gallbladder disease is 3 times more common in women than men; symptoms occur between the ages of 35 and 55 years. The existence of stones does not mean that surgery must be performed. Many people have stones, but the stones have not collected in areas where they cause pain or obstruction. However, the majority of persons so afflicted probably will develop symptoms related to indigestion: gas, heartburn, bloating, nausea and pain. Sometimes the pain is knifelike in the upper right part of the abdomen, and often it is shooting to the back or the right shoulder region.

The acute pain is the result of one or more of the stones getting caught in the small cystic duct. When food is being digested, a chemical action causes the gallbladder to contract and force its contents into the cystic duct, then the common bile duct, and finally into the intestine. When the narrow cystic duct is obstructed because of a stone, one of three things may happen: (1) the stone can drop back into the gallbladder, and the attack subsides; (2) the stone can continue to block the duct and produce inflammation and infection which may demand immediate surgery, or (3) the stone can pass into the common bile duct. Once in the common bile duct, the stone either will pass into the intestine or be caught in the duct near the exit point at the intestine. When the latter situation occurs, the flow of bile is obstructed, and the patient develops jaundice (yellow-green discoloration of the skin and possibly the cornea). Immediate surgery is necessary in this situation. Not only must the stone-bearing gallbladder be removed, but the common bile duct also must be cleared by either lifting out the stone (with a stone forceps) or incising the duct at the point of obstruction and delivering it.

The Operation

The patient is placed in a supine position on the operating table in such a way that the gallbladder region is directly above the kidney rest, which later may be elevated to hyperextend that area for better exposure.

The patient is given a general anesthetic, his skin is prepared, and he is draped. Usually, a subcostal incision is made in the upper right quadrant. After meticulous layer-by-layer dissection (fat, muscle, aponeuroses) and maintaining hemostasis, the surgeon incises the peritoneum to expose the cavity and the liver. The liver is elevated and retracted to permit visualization of the gallbladder.

At this point one or more of the following procedures will be undertaken:

1. If a *cholangiogram* (x-ray picture of the biliary tract) is ordered, the dye is injected by a syringe, and x-ray pictures are taken. Warm, moist sponges protect the viscera during exploration.

2. If the gallbladder is to be removed, the surgeon gently dissects it free from its liver bed. When this is accomplished, the cystic duct is clamped with two special clamps. The duct is severed, and the gallbladder is removed.

3. If the gallbladder is to be drained, a trocar pierces the gallbladder, and its bile is suctioned. The surgeon examines the gallbladder for stones, which he lifts out or scoops out with appropriate instruments. Usually, a rubber drain is inserted and held in place with a purse-string suture.

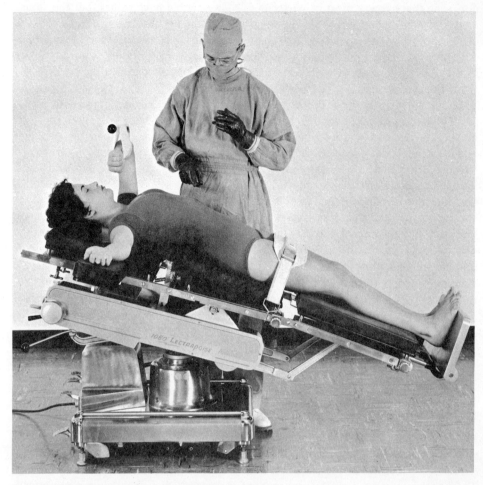

Fig. 101. This model is demonstrating the position used for operations on the gallbladder.
Note the elevation of the table and the mattress at the subcostal region where
the gallbladder is located. Also note that the head end of the table is elevated.
(AMSCO, American Sterilizer Company, Erie, Pa.)

4. If the common bile duct is to be examined for obstruction or drained, special
probes, catheters and forceps will be used. Following this a T-tube will be inserted
into the common duct to give strength and support during healing. This tube is
used also to determine visibly the postoperative flow of bile from the liver, since it
will be connected to a drainage tubing and bottle when the patient returns to his
bed. In 4 to 6 days the T-tube is removed.

Following the sponge count and careful accounting for instruments and needles,
the abdomen is closed in the usual manner of layer-by-layer approximation. The
T-tube is fastened carefully, and the final dressing is applied.

Fig. 102. Diagram of a T-tube in place
after choledochostomy.

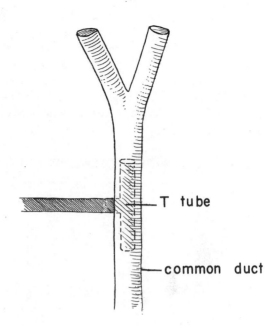

T tube

common   duct

GASTRECTOMY

This term means removal of the stomach (gastro = stomach; ectomy = removal of). Removal of only a portion of the stomach is called a subtotal gastrectomy.

THE STOMACH

The stomach is a relatively small part of the alimentary tract (digestive system), which is a continuous tubular structure about 28 feet long, beginning at the mouth and ending at the anus. A normal empty stomach measures about 8 inches in length and is about 4 inches wide. It is a highly muscular bag that is located in the upper abdomen on the left side in the epigastric region (Fig. 103) just below the broad muscular band called the diaphragm and extending to the right of the midline.

The upper end of the stomach, where the esophagus enters, is called the cardiac end. The lower end, where the stomach enters into the small intestine (duodenem), is called the pyloric region. Guarding this junction is a muscular ring of tissue (sphincter) that, acting like a valve, opens and closes, regulating the flow of food out of the stomach. A congenital problem affecting some infants is a narrowing of this valve, a condition called pyloric stenosis. Figure 103 shows two other landmarks commonly referred to as the greater and the lesser curvatures of the stomach.

Functions. The stomach is a storehouse for food. Since it is a muscular sac, it can expand and contract as necessary. Large amounts of food can be received and then released by degrees when the rest of the digestive system is ready for it.

Part of the digestive process takes place in the stomach. Peristalsis, a rhythmic contraction of muscles, provides a mechanical churning motion while the food is in the stomach. This process is combined with a chemical breakdown of foods. The walls of the stomach are lined with small glands that secrete gastric juice and hydrochloric acid. The gastric juice contains two enzymes that act on proteins and break them into simpler forms. Hydrochloric acid kills bacteria that enter the stomach with food, and it also helps to regulate the opening and the closing of the pyloric valve. Following this chemical and mechanical action, food leaves the stomach in a semiliquid form. Further digestive processes take place beyond the stomach in the small intestine.

Surgical Treatment of Stomach Disorders

Ulcers. The most common reason for performing surgery in this area is the presence of a duodenal ulcer. The duodenum (about 10 inches long) is the beginning

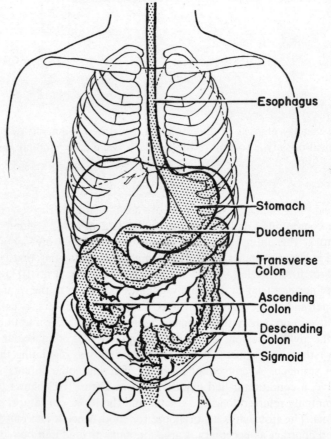

Fig. 103. Diagram showing the position of the digestive organs. (Emerson, P. E., Jr., and Bragdon, J. S.: Essentials of Medicine, ed. 18, p. 518, Philadelphia, Lippincott, 1959)

of the small intestine and is attached to the stomach at the pylorus. It is a common site of ulceration, which is a weakening of tissue walls to form a raw surface and an inflamed base (much like a sore). A large percentage of duodenal ulcers and of gastric ulcers (ulcers that develop in the stomach proper) can be healed under conservative medical management without surgery. When surgery is indicated, generally medical treatment has failed, and hyperacidity (the formation of excessive amounts of acid secretions) continues.

The surgical procedure is designed to remove that portion of the stomach and the duodenum containing acid-secreting glands. The surgeon may remove from 60 to 80 per cent of the stomach and about 2 inches of the duodenum. After tightly closing the duodenum stump, he re-establishes the continuity of the tract by suturing the remainder of the stomach to the jejunum (second part of the small intestine). This joining is called an *anastomosis*. (Fig. 104)

After this operation food passes to the new sac formed by joining the remnants of the stomach to the small intestine. The patient is advised to have limited food intake for about 4 months, after which time the sac distends, and he can eat normally. For the majority of patients this surgery is successful. A small number of patients have a recurrence of symptoms, and a *vagotomy* is performed. In this operation the vagus nerve, the main nerve supplying the stomach wall, is severed. After this procedure most patients are cured of symptoms.

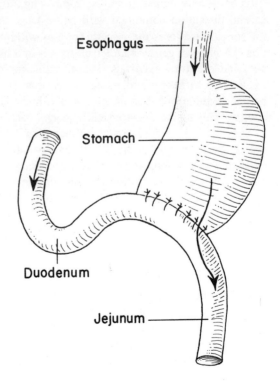

Fig. 104. One type of anastomosis.

An immediate operation is necessary when an ulcer perforates (breaks through the wall), forming a hole, with the contents of the organ bathing internal tissues. A patient with a perforated ulcer is acutely ill and usually in shock. An emergency operation is done to close the hole (plication). More extensive surgery at this time might further threaten the patient's life. Although a gastrectomy might be done at a later date, many of these patients do not require a second operation.

Tumors of the stomach are more common in men than in women. Careful x-ray studies confirm the presence of pathology, but only surgical excision can confirm the diagnosis. There are many benign (noncancerous) tumors of the stomach, i.e., polyps, fatty tumors, muscle tumors. Removal of these tumors usually results in permanent recovery. Malignant tumors of the stomach also can be cured if they are treated in the early stages of the condition. A subtotal or a total gastrectomy may be necessary, in which is used a modification of the operation described for the surgical treatment of gastric or duodenal ulcer.

Gastrectomy. This operation is a major surgical procedure which often takes 3 to 5 hours to complete, depending on the complexities encountered. The patient is placed in supine position (flat on his back). The anesthetic is usually either general inhalation anesthesia or spinal. Careful accounting of gauze sponges is vital, since the abdominal cavity will be entered. Following meticulous antisepsis of the skin, the application of sterile drapes and the connection of sterile suction equipment, the surgeon usually makes either an upper longitudinal or a left oblique incision. After careful dissection combined with hemostasis, the peritoneal cavity is entered, and the surgeon explores the viscera (organs within the cavity). Throughout the operation the surgeon gently handles all tissues and uses a variety of absorbable and nonabsorbable suture materials. Warm saline-moistened sponges are used to protect tissues and to keep them moist. A number of specialized instruments are used to prevent trauma of the stomach and the intestine and to avoid spillage of intestinal content. During the anastomosis a special gastrointestinal technic often is employed to protect surrounding tissues. When this is done, selected instruments are not reused or returned to the sterile Mayo stand. Regowning and regloving of the surgeon and his assistant often are necessary after the anastomosis has been completed. During the operation the patient is given blood and other intravenous fluids to prevent surgical shock. A stomach tube usually is passed to keep the tract empty postoperatively and to permit healing to take place. After the first postoperative day, early ambulation is encouraged. The convalescent period for most patients takes about 8 weeks.

HEMORRHOIDS AND OTHER RECTAL PROBLEMS

In adults the last 5 to 6 inches of the gastrointestinal tract is referred to as the *rectum;* the last inch of rectum is called the *anus.* This outlet is made up of muscle bands which expand and contract with the passage of each stool. This muscle is called a *sphincter.* The anus is very sensitive and can cause discomfort if it is cleaned improperly, or if irregularity is a problem. (Fig. 105)

Fig. 105. External and internal hemorrhoids. (Brunner, L. S., *et al.*: Medical-Surgical Nursing, p. 640, Philadelphia, Lippincott, 1964)

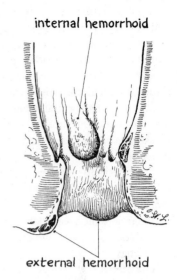

internal hemorrhoid

external hemorrhoid

CONDITIONS OF THE LOWER INTESTINAL TRACT

Many people claim that their general feeling of well-being is related directly to proper bowel function. Symptoms which cause concern are chronic constipation, rectal itching, bleeding, persistent diarrhea or hemorrhoids (piles).

Hemorrhoids occur when the veins which drain the rectal and the anal regions become stretched and dilated, a condition which may occur with repeated stress during defecation. Gravity also imposes a strain on these veins, and any abdominal pressure increases it. This may occur in laborers who lift heavy loads, in fighter pilots who are subjected to great pressures in their abdominal organs, and even in military men who ride over rough terrain. Chronic constipation, mental and emotional stress, and pregnancy also may contribute to the formation of hemorrhoids.

These engorged vessels are varicose veins, and their treatment may not require an operation. Relief may be obtained by medication (codeine and aspirin), bed rest, hot or cold compresses to the anus, sitz baths, mineral oil orally, and the application of an anesthetic ointment or spray locally. However, if the weakened blood vessels become inflamed or infected, they may need surgery. Often, the irritation that results from repeated contraction and expansion during bowel evacuation is sufficient to cause ulcers and hemorrhage. When such a vessel becomes inflamed, the condition is called *phlebitis,* and if a clot also is formed, the condition is referred to as *thrombosed hemorrhoids.* Such hemorrhoids may become enlarged and push out externally as painful lumps.

Treatment. INJECTION. Internal hemorrhoids may be treated by injecting them with a sclerosing solution, such as quinine-urea-hydrochloride, instilled into the submucosal layer of the rectum. This produces an inflammatory reaction, followed by the formation of hard, fibrous tissue, which in turn causes the vessels to shrink.

This procedure is done with the patient in the endoscopy (knee-chest) position, and the anoscope in position. As the scope is withdrawn, each hemorrhoid that comes into view is injected. Injection of hemorrhoids is not considered to be a cure but rather a temporary measure.

SURGICAL EXCISION is the preferred method of treating prolapsed internal hemorrhoids, internal combined with external hemorrhoids, or strangulated hemorrhoids. Symptoms which usually herald such difficulties are protrusion, pain and bleeding. The clot may be removed by first infiltrating the area with a local anesthetic; then the mass may be incised, or an elliptical incision may be made over the clot, and it can be expressed.

The anesthetic chosen is one that combats muscular spasm and gives the greatest relaxation. Favorite methods are *saddle block* or *caudal* anesthesia. In saddle block a local anesthetic is injected into the lower spine (blocking pain in the lower body area which ordinarily would touch a saddle). In caudal the area of the cauda equina nerves, which spray out of the spinal cord like hairs of a horse's tail, is injected with procaine or metycaine which anesthetizes the lower abdominal area.

The patient is placed in the lithotomy (legs up in stirrups) position on the operating table. Drapes are applied to cover the legs and to allow adequate perineal exposure. (See p. 160.) Other positions which can be used are Sims's lateral, jackknife, Kraske, etc.

After the surrounding skin and rectal mucosa have been washed to make the area as surgically clean as possible, a rectal speculum is inserted to expose the internal varicosities. Each hemorrhoid is grasped with a toothed instrument. The tissue directly over the hemorrhoid is incised, veins are dissected, and bleeders are tied. The base of the hemorrhoid then is tied with a transfixion suture, and the hemorrhoid distal to the ligation is cut free. Some surgeons prefer to use a special hemorrhoid clamp to anchor the hemorrhoid during its excision.

Postoperatively, a small rubber drain or wick of petrolatum gauze may be inserted through the sphincter to allow drainage of blood. Dressings may or may not be used.

Other Rectal Conditions. *Fissure in ano* is an ulcer of the rectum that is best described as a cracklike opening in the anal canal. It does not heal readily since it is repeatedly irritated by the passage of hard stool. This causes a spasm of the rectal sphincter, and the patient has severe pain. Often the patient has a tendency to constipation, because he attempts to avoid defecation and the resulting pain. There are several ways to treat an anal fissure. Sometimes it will heal following dilatation; or the fissure may be excised. In some instances the external sphincter is divided, producing partial paralysis of the sphincter but relieving the spasm and permitting the ulcer to heal. (Fig. 106)

Fistula in ano is a tiny tunnellike opening which leads from the skin near the anus through a tortuous path to the rectal canal. Pus leaks from the opening, necessitating the wearing of a pad. This condition can be repaired in the operating room after the surgeon has identified the tract by inserting a probe or injecting a dye,

Fig. 106. (*Top*) Fissure in ano. (*Bottom*) Fistula in ano. (Brunner, L. S., *et al.:* Medical - Surgical Nursing, p. 640, Philadelphia, Lippincott, 1964)

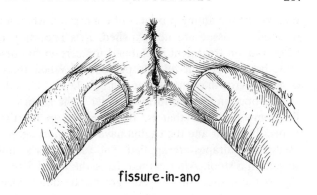

fissure-in-ano

hypertrophied papilla

fistula

methylene blue, into the external opening. The fistula is then cut open and packed with gauze. (Fig. 106)

D. AND C. OPERATION

These letters mean dilatation (stretching) of the cervix, and curettage (scraping) of the uterine lining. The procedure is either diagnostic to determine the cause of various gynecologic disorders or therapeutic.

As a diagnostic procedure, tissue specimens of the uterine lining (endometrium) are processed and microscopically evaluated to determine whether an abnormal growth is developing within the uterus; the reasons for disturbance of the regular menstrual flow with either excessive bleeding or failure to menstruate; or the causes of sterility (inability to become pregnant).

A D. and C. also may be a therapeutic procedure. For instance, it is employed to remove the remaining products of conception when a women has had a miscarriage; if shreds of tissue are not expelled, it is necessary to clean out the cavity. Also, when radium treatment is planned for certain tumors of the uterus, the lining first must be cleaned out by this procedure. When there are polyps (tabs of tissue) or an overgrowth of the uterine lining, a D. and C. is done.

The operation is performed under light general anesthesia with the patient in lithotomy position (that is, the legs are up in stirrups—leg-holders). After the pubis, the thighs and the vagina have been thoroughly washed, rinsed and antiseptics used, sterile drapes are applied. The surgeon is scrubbed, gowned and gloved, and seated on a stool. After catheterizing the bladder to remove all urine, which would distort the tissues, the surgeon grasps the outer edge of the cervix and brings the organ forward. A weighted retractor depresses the posterior wall of the vagina. Having determined the depth and the position of the uterus, the surgeon uses size-graduated dilators temporarily to expand the cervical os (opening). A long gauze sponge is placed on the blade of the weighted retractor as the surgeon, in a careful clockwise manner, uses long slender curettes to begin the clean-out process. As he scrapes, blood and tissue collect on the sponge. When the uterus is clean, a characteristic "hollow" sound usually can be heard.

Note: Care must be taken to insure that *all* tissue immediately is placed into a fixative so that shreds will not dehydrate or distort before the pathologist can evaluate them.

In placing the patient in lithotomy position and at the completion of the procedure another person should assist in handling the legs so that undue strain on the muscles of the pelvis or the legs can be avoided.

No external incision is made, and the operation causes very little discomfort.

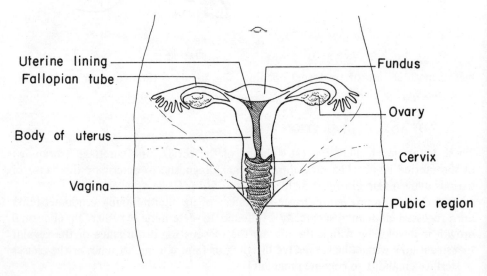

Fig. 107. Diagrammatic view of the female reproductive organs.

Fig. 108. Schematic drawing of urinary tract.

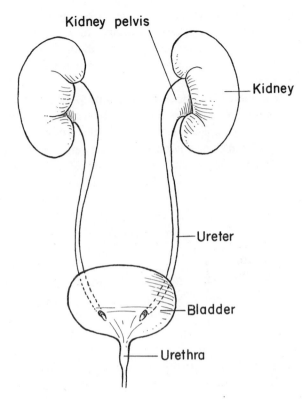

Kidney pelvis

Kidney

Ureter

Bladder

Urethra

The patient leaves the operating room with a perineal pad in place to absorb drainage. This procedure causes the patient to be incapacitated for only 1 or 2 days.

CYSTOSCOPY

A *cystoscopy* is an examination of the urinary bladder through a metal, lens-carrying instrument called a cystoscope. As was described on page 70, the construction of this instrument permits visualization of the interior wall of the bladder. A *cystoscopic examination* is a diagnostic procedure indicated for patients with hematuria (blood in urine), urinary tract obstruction, or calculi (stones).

Most hospitals set aside a room for these procedures located just outside the operating room suite or near the x-ray department. These locations are desirable since many of these patients are evaluated as outpatients. A special cystoscopy table is used. It is equipped with drainage troughs and permits x-ray pictures to be taken concurrent with the procedure.

Every effort is made by doctors and nurses to explain the procedure to the patient to allay his fears and gain his cooperation. Most of these patients are examined under local anesthesia, although a general anesthetic may be given when more extensive work is necessary, or when the patient is unduly apprehensive. Fluids are encouraged before the patient goes to the cystoscopy room to insure a continuous flow of urine in the event that samples of urine may be necessary from the kidneys.

The patient is placed in lithotomy position on the cystoscopy table, and care is taken to avoid pressure points. The operative area is cleaned thoroughly, and sterile drapes are applied, leaving only the perineum exposed. (Preoperative shaving usually is not considered to be necessary for this procedure.) Local anesthesia is instilled into the urethra immediately before the cystoscope is inserted. Usually, the scope is passed easily; asking the patient to breathe deeply often will relax muscle spasms. Once the instrument is in place, the bladder is filled with distilled water to distend it and permit visualization of the tissues.

Frequently, it is necessary for the surgeon to pass x-ray-detectable ureteral catheters through the scope, threading them into the ureteral bladder openings. The catheters are passed up the ureters into the kidney pelvis (Fig. 108). Urine specimens are taken from one or both kidneys as a part of such a ureteral catheterization. These specimens usually are examined microscopically, cultured, and studied for the presence of cancer cells or tuberculosis. Kidney function tests often are performed. After intravenous injection of a dye into the arm of the patient, the physician will time the appearance of the dye from each kidney. When the kidneys are functioning normally, the dye appears in 3 to 6 minutes.

When it is necessary to visualize the kidney and the ureters, an x-ray-detectable substance is instilled within the ureteral catheters to outline the kidneys. X-ray pictures are taken, and as the scope and the catheters are removed, more dye is introduced to outline the ureters. Again, more x-ray pictures are taken. This examination is called a *retrograde pyelogram.*

These important diagnostic examinations require no external incision. It must be remembered that the apprehension of a patient undergoing such examinations usually is great. Extreme tact and understanding must be shown by all personnel who assist in the procedure.

Cystoscopes and catheters should be sterilized for these procedures. When equipment to accomplish this is lacking, careful disinfection technics must be followed.

VEIN LIGATION AND STRIPPING

These operations are concerned with the cutting and ligation (tying off) of veins and/or the stripping—literally pulling off—of the main branch of a vein.

Varicose veins, also called varicosities, are herniations or outpockets of parts of veins due to sectional weakness or breakdown. The function of the veins is to return blood from body tissues to the heart and the lungs. The heart does the work of pumping blood through the body. Other important help comes from the contraction of muscles in the body. The presence of one-way valves in the venous system prevents blood from running backward. (Fig. 109)

When valves are defective, varicosities occur, because the inadequately drained tissue becomes susceptible to infection. This often happens in obesity as well as in pregnancy. Unusual pressure on the veins in the pelvis may bring pressure on the veins in the thigh and the legs. Dentists, sales clerks, barbers and others who stand in one position for long periods of time often suffer from varicosities. Muscle action helps to return blood, and prolonged muscle inactivity puts a greater strain on the valves. Damage to the valves then follows, causing vessels to dilate and blood to stagnate within them. Inflammation within veins (phlebitis) also may cause destruction of valves and result in varicosities.

Fortunately, this condition usually is limited to involvement of the superficial veins under the skin rather than the deep veins which carry the bulk of the blood of the body back to the heart. It is for this reason that after surgery for varicose veins the blood that formerly stagnated in veins can move to the efficient deep vessels to return to the heart. Infrequently, deep veins are obstructed because of previous phlebitis. When this occurs, the superficial vessels would not be tied off or stripped.

One of the most succesful treatments for varicose veins is to ligate and cut the main saphenous vein and all of its branches in the groin. This procedure changes the course of venous blood flow from the superficial veins to the deep veins of the legs and the thighs.

When the surgeon believes that there are sluggish valves connecting superficial and deep veins in the whole extremity, he often decides to make additional multiple incisions in the thighs or the legs to cut and ligate the vessel along the course of the varicosities. When this decision is made, the patient will be asked to stand erect for a short time to permit the blood supply to pool, while the surgeon, using a skin-marking pencil, outlines the points of the varicosities which later will be incised.

Vein ligation operations usually are performed under spinal or local anesthesia. The extremity is washed carefully with antibacterial soap, and antiseptics are used. Sterile drapes are applied by the surgeon, and the operation begins. The surgeon dissects carefully to find the right vessel and its branches, which are cut and tied. Although this operation is not considered to be dangerous to the patient's life, meticulous surgery generally requires that 1 or 2 hours be taken to complete the case. A snug bandage is applied to the extremity after surgery, and the patient is encouraged to walk soon after the operation.

LIGATION AND STRIPPING OF THE MAIN SAPHENOUS VEIN

For extensive varicosities some surgeons believe that multiple incisions to cut and ligate the vessel do not provide a cure. These surgeons perform a stripping of the main saphenous vein. To accomplish this, a long slender wire (vein stripper) is threaded through the main vessel in the groin and pushed through along the course of the vein to the ankle. An incision is made over the ankle, and the wire

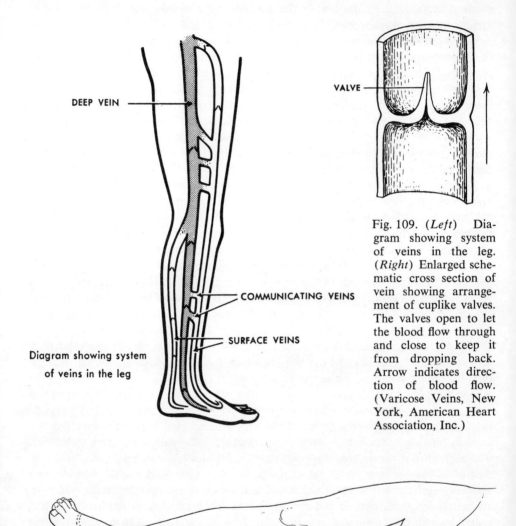

DEEP VEIN

VALVE

COMMUNICATING VEINS

SURFACE VEINS

Diagram showing system
of veins in the leg

Fig. 109. (*Left*)   Diagram showing system
of veins in the leg.
(*Right*) Enlarged sche-
matic cross section of
vein showing arrange-
ment of cuplike valves.
The valves open to let
the blood flow through
and close to keep it
from dropping back.
Arrow indicates direc-
tion of blood flow.
(Varicose Veins, New
York, American Heart
Association, Inc.)

Stripper emerging from vein
at ankle

Vein stripper
in saphenous vein

Fig. 110. Stripping the main saphenous vein. The vein stripper is threaded through the
main vessel in the groin and pushed through along the course of the vein to the
ankle. An incision is made over the ankle, and the wire is grasped.

is grasped. In the groin the wire is tied securely to the vein, and then the wire is pulled out from the ankle. This maneuver permits the vein to be removed from above downward by inversion within itself (inside out). (Fig. 110)

Although there is a high rate of cure with this operation, the complications of hemorrhage beneath the skin and sometimes infection are not infrequent.

ORTHOPEDIC SURGERY

Orthopedics is that branch of surgery which deals with the prevention or the correction of deformities, the repair of traumatic injuries, and the treatment of diseases of bones, joints, ligaments, cartilage, tendons, muscles and nerves associated with the skeletal framework of the body.

Congenital deformities (defects present at birth), fortunately are rare, and modern treatment can markedly benefit patients with clubfoot, dislocated hip, or extra fingers or toes. Even more rare are deformities resulting in the absence of an extremity. Such tragedies usually are attributed to some failure in intra-uterine development. Injury incurred while the embryo (developing baby) is growing in the uterus may result in torticollis (wryneck) or in deformities of the spine. Non-operative, continuous treatment beginning at birth has shown good results. Surgery is done on a small number of such cases in which conservative treatment has failed.

There are a number of complex orthopedic operations which require special study and supervised experience on the part of the nursing assistant or technician if she is to be of competent assistance to the surgical team. However, the more common problems are associated with fractures.

DEFINITION AND CLASSIFICATION OF A FRACTURE

A fracture is a break in the continuity of bone. Considering that there are over 200 bones in the body, it is understandable that a fracture of one or more bones in a lifetime is a probability. Fractures may occur as a result of a direct or an indirect injury by a slip, a fall, a severe wrench, or from a slight injury in a patient whose bones may be weakened by disease.

The two main classifications of fractures are *simple* and *compound*. A *simple* fracture is a break in a bone without a break in the skin surface. A *compound* fracture is a break in a bone that communicates with the exterior of the body through a break in the skin. The distinction between the two types is important, because infection and delayed healing are much greater when the fracture is compound.

Fractures are further classified according to position, number and shape of bone fragments as being transverse, serrated, comminuted, greenstick, multiple, etc. Figure 111 shows these classifications. (See also Fig: 112.)

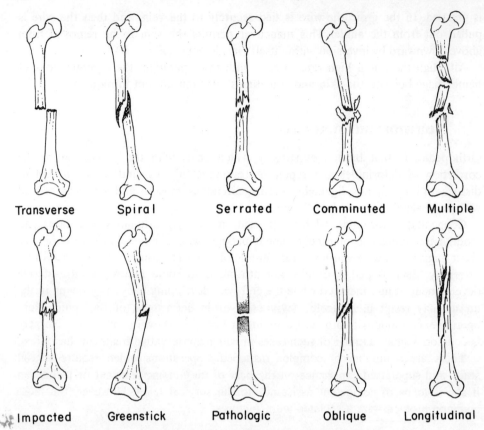

Transverse   Spiral   Serrated   Comminuted   Multiple

Impacted   Greenstick   Pathologic   Oblique   Longitudinal

Fig. 111. Classification of fractures. (Adapted from Department of the Army, Medical and Surgical Technicians, TM 8-230, 1961)

DIAGNOSIS OF A FRACTURE

The physician makes the diagnosis of a fracture by first evaluating the patient's symptoms. These may include hearing or feeling a bone snap, pain and tenderness, partial or complete loss of function, deformity, swelling and dislocation, appearance of bone fragments. X-ray pictures then are taken to confirm the diagnosis and to determine the amount of damage to the bone and to other bones in the area.

FACTORS NECESSARY FOR GOOD HEALING OF BONE

These are:

1. The condition of the patient, his age and his state of nutrition. Bone repairs itself more readily in young persons than in the elderly; bones become brittle with

aging, because the aging process causes a higher proportion of minerals to be deposited in the bones.

2. Good circulation to both fragments of the fracture.

3. Proper immobilization (placing the part at rest) with no soft tissue or muscle between bone ends and with good "locking" and alignment.

4. Absence of infection.

5. Formation of osteoblasts (bone-forming cells), which grow in from the periosteum (thin membranous bone covering) to replace soft callus, which first forms about the margin of the break. Osteoblasts turn soft callus into hard callus to form union.

Fixation of Fractures

Whether there is a simple or a compound fracture, the bone fractures must be *reduced* ("set" properly in place). This is accomplished by either *open* or *closed* reduction.

Closed reduction is a manipulation of the extremity, usually under a light anesthesia, followed by application of a splint or a cast. This procedure often is done in an emergency room or cast room, where cast equipment as well as suction and oxygen are present.

Open reduction is a major operation with incision over the site of fracture, visual exposure and reduction of the fracture, often with internal fixation with wire, screws, nails or plates. These procedures are done in surgery under strict aseptic conditions. It often is necessary to use a special orthopedic table to replace the standard operating room table. Orthopedic tables and their accessories are designed to afford maximum assistance to the surgeon in positioning and operating on patients. Extreme care is exercised and a number of assistants are used to move the patient onto the table without further damage to the affected part.

The skin is prepared carefully and draped. Because sterile adherent plastic drapes (see Fig. 41) conform well to the extremities, they often are incorporated in the draping procedure. However, wide stockinette and multiple sheets also may be used. The incision is made over the injured area, and bleeding vessels are clamped and tied. Layer by layer the tissues are cut or divided until good exposure of the broken bone is obtained. A variety of special instruments may be necessary in the repair and the reduction of the bone. Some of these tools resemble those which may be found in a carpenter's workshop, i.e., screws, screwdrivers, chisels, gouges, drills, bits and hammers. The surgeon previously will have alerted the operating room supervisor regarding the fixation equipment he will need. All of the objects should be sterilized for the procedure. To avoid undue tissue reaction, care must be taken by all personnel to assure that any screws and plates used during the operation are made of the same metal—i.e., stainless steel or vitallium. The patient's previous x-ray pictures are mounted in the room to assist the surgeon further in obtaining good alignment. It often is advisable to repeat x-ray pictures before the closure of

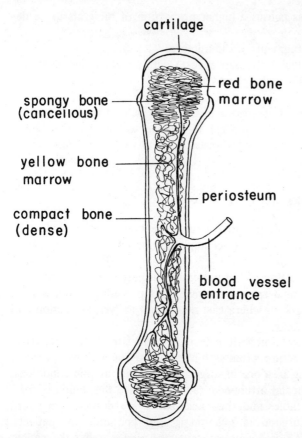

cartilage

Fig. 112. Cross-sectional diagram of a long bone.

red bone
marrow

spongy bone
(cancellous)

yellow bone
marrow

compact bone
(dense)

periosteum

blood vessel
entrance

the wound. When the operation involves entrance into a deep wound, as in the repair of a fractured hip, sponge counts are made by nursing personnel. (Figs. 113, 114)

APPLICATION OF CAST

When it is necessary to immobilize a patient's leg, arm, or body, a plaster cast may be applied. Operating room personnel prepare the equipment and supplies and assist the surgeon in the application of cast materials. If a portable plaster cart is to be used, it is wheeled into the operating room. If the room is a specialized orthopedic room, the necessary supplies and equipment are stored in a built-in cabinet or closet. Commercially available plaster of Paris is a chalky white powder impregnated within strips of crinoline of various widths. The strips are rolled in convenient lengths and are wrapped individually to prevent the powder from separating from the crinoline. When a roll of plaster is placed in water, a chemical process of rehydration (restoration of water content to a substance which has been dehydrated) takes place. This generates a small amount of heat, which makes the cast feel warm to the patient as it sets.

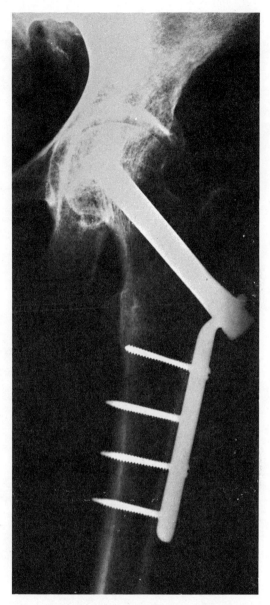

Fig. 113. (*Top*) X-ray picture showing fixation with a plate and screws intact. (*Bottom*) Fixation plate with screw holes.

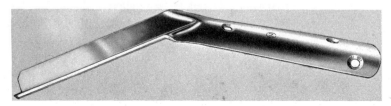

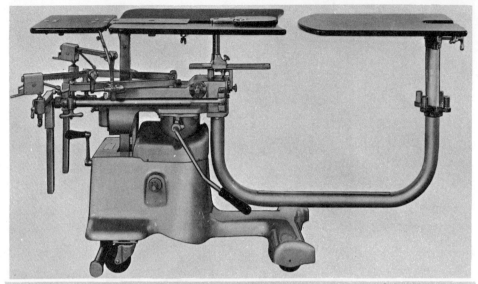

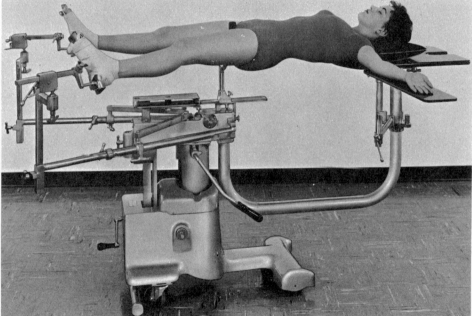

Fig. 114. (*Top*) Albee orthopedic operating table. (*Bottom*) Albee table illustrating the positioning of a patient. (AMSCO, American Sterilizer Company, Erie, Pa.)

A lined plaster pail is filled with water that is tepid rather than hot. Hot water may cause loss of plaster from the roll, and it also increases the setting time. The furniture and the floor should be protected from plaster splashes by lengths of disposable paper or plastic sheeting. Every effort should be made to avoid getting deposits of plaster on linen sheets or drapes, because it is difficult to wash off, and it can clog ordinary laundry drains.

The surgeon cuts and fits felt or foam padding to protect the skin and bony prominences, or he may use stockinette and sheet wadding for this purpose. Wide edges are left below and above the areas of the cast so that they later may be sealed to prevent plaster crumbs from gathering under the cast and causing irritation to the skin. When the surgeon is ready to apply the cast, the assistant takes a roll of the designated width, holding it with both hands, one on either end of the roll. The plaster roll then is submerged below the water level and held about 5 to 10 seconds until air bubbles are released. The roll then is removed from the water and is squeezed *gently* at both ends, a maneuver which removes a great deal of the water but leaves the roll well moistened.

This softened roll is handed to the surgeon with the free end readily apparent. He applies this and subsequent rolls with turns overlapping to create a strong, even cast. The plaster rolls are prepared one at a time as they are needed; if they were to be prepared far in advance of need, they would harden and have to be discarded. If accessories are needed, such as a crossbar or a walking caliper (iron), the surgeon will indicate when he is ready to incorporate them into the cast.

An assistant may be asked to support the extremity as a cast is being applied. The surgeon determines the position and the amount of traction (if any) required to maintain proper bone alignment. Holding must be done as directed with gentle but steady pressure, using the palms of the hands rather than the fingers. By providing a cradle of support, finger pressure imprints on the cast can be avoided.

As the cast is completed, the surgeon turns a cuff of stockinette or sheet wadding over the raw edges of the cast and anchors them with the last few turns of the plaster roll. This seals the plaster edges and provides a smooth neat finish to the cast. Excess plaster on the patient's skin, fingers or toes should be removed before the plaster sets. Note that toes and fingers were deliberately exposed to provide a means of checking the adequacy of circulation.

Pillows with rubber or plastic covering may be used to support the extremity until it is thoroughly air-dried. Depending on the type of plaster used, the drying period may take from 5 minutes to several hours.

REVIEW QUESTIONS:
1. Since bleeding may be a problem during or after a tonsillectomy, what equipment should be available, and how is it used?
2. What is a frozen section, and why is it done? If you are scrubbed, and a frozen section is done, what is involved when the laboratory report is positive? If negative?

3. What precautions must be taken when the stump of an appendix is cauterized? Why?
4. When the common bile duct is explored, what additional sterile supplies will be needed by the scrubbed assistant that are not needed for a cholecystectomy? Indicate the purpose for these additions.
5. What is meant by anastomosis? Give an example.
6. Differentiate: fistula in ano, fissure in ano, hemorrhoid.
7. Why and how is a dilatation and curettage performed?
8. List the differences between an abdominal operation and a cystoscopy.
9. What is the difference between vein ligation and stripping of a vein for varicose veins?
10. What do you need and how would you assist a surgeon in applying a cast to a patient's leg?

Bibliography

Alexander, E. L.: Care of the Patient in Surgery, St. Louis, Mosby, 1958.
Hall, E. D.: Surgical Instrument Guide for Nurses, Brooklyn, N.Y., Weck, 1954.
Manual of Operative Procedure and Surgical Knots, Somerville, N.J., Ethicon, Inc., 1961.
Nursing Care of the Patient in Ob-Gyn Surgery, Somerville, N.J., Ethicon, Inc., 1964.
Nursing Care of the Patient in Orthopaedic Surgery, Somerville, N.J., Ethicon, Inc., 1965.

UNIT **5**

Postoperative Care

CHAPTER **12**

CARE OF THE PATIENT, THE OPERATING ROOM AND EQUIPMENT FOLLOWING SURGERY

CARE OF THE PATIENT : CARE OF ROOM, EQUIPMENT, SUPPLIES
AND INSTRUMENTS

CARE OF THE PATIENT

THE END OF THE OPERATION

When the last suture has been tied and cut, and the incision has been closed, the surgeon cleans the area around the incision and uses a chemical antiseptic or spray such as PVP (see Chap. 4, p. 64). After the skin is dry, the scrub assistant hands him sterile dressings, which he applies. He holds the dressings in place while the drapes are removed, and the circulating nurse assists him with the application of adhesive tape or other needed dressing supplies. Exposure of the patient should be minimal.

The administration of anesthesia may have been discontinued shortly before this. The anesthetist makes his final evaluation of the patient's condition and asks the surgeon for orders on the administration of I.V. fluids, blood, or other indicated therapy.

The patient's gown is changed if it is soiled or damp, and then he is transferred to a special stretcher equipped with side guards, receptacles for intravenous poles, and wheel brakes. It also is designed to assume Trendelenburg and reverse Trendelenburg positions easily and quickly. Wheel brakes on the stretcher and on the wheels of the operating room table should be locked when the patient is being

233

moved from one to the other. The orderly may be called to help to transfer the patient, although it is customary for all members of the team to assist in this. The anesthetist controls the head and the neck of the patient, who is moved only with the anesthetist's approval. A simple and easy method of transferring a patient from the operating table to the stretcher is to use a patient roller (Fig. 115). This device allows the patient to be moved with no strain on him or the personnel. The anesthetist and the circulating nurse or the orderly takes the patient and his chart to the recovery room.

THE RECOVERY ROOM

The anesthetist gives the recovery room nurse pertinent information about the patient, his operative course, his present condition and postoperative orders. Although he leaves the recovery room, the anesthetist remains immediately available if the nurses should require his assistance.

The recovery room nurse observes and notes the kind and the type of drainage to be used, if any (such as low-level Wangensteen continuous suction for thoracic drainage), the condition of the dressings, and the amount of bleeding. Vital signs (blood pressure, pulse and respirations) are checked and recorded every 5 minutes until stabilized, and then every 15 minutes for 2 hours. Condition of skin, signs of shock or hemorrhage, respiratory difficulty or other serious symptoms indicate the immediate need for evaluation by a physician. He is summoned by the recovery room nurse.

Recovery room personnel are specially trained to assist the patient in his return to normal function as safely and comfortably as possible. Emphasis is placed on the prevention of complications. The judgment, the education and the experience of the recovery room nurse enable her to assess patient condition intelligently. When ominous signs occur, she recognizes the problem quickly and institutes immediate relief.

The equipment available in the recovery room is designed for particular conditions that might arise. Aids for breathing (oxygen, tracheotomy sets, laryngoscopes, etc.), circulation (sphygmomanometers, I.V. trays, cutdown sets, etc.), sterile dressings and emergency drugs are kept available.

The recovery room like the operating room is kept clean, quiet and orderly. The walls are painted in muted soft colors. Indirect lighting illuminates the room, though high-intensity lighting also is available for treatments, examinations, etc. Equipment is arranged conveniently for use, with space and facilities provided for needs in the work areas.

The surgeon visits his patient in the recovery room at intervals, and he or some other physician is available at all times for emergencies that might arise.

The anesthesiologist or a member of the anesthesia staff discharges the patient from the recovery room (usually in writing), to be returned to the patient unit when the patient's condition indicates that he is ready.

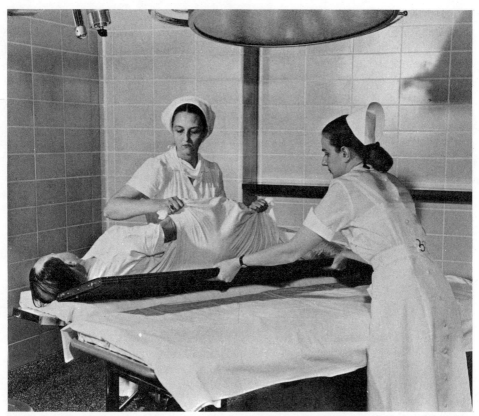

Fig. 115. The lightweight roller with a black conductive cover aids in moving the patient with minimum effort and maximum comfort. (Davis patient roller, Gilbert Hyde Chick Company, Oakland, Calif.)

CARE OF SPECIMENS

The pathology laboratory in each hospital usually specifies the fixative solution to be used on specimens and the manner of delivery to the laboratory. Some prefer sending one of their laboratory personnel to the operating room 2 or 3 times a day to pick up the specimens. In a hospital with fewer operations each day, the pickup may be only once a day in the midafternoon. In other institutions the operating room may be responsible for sending the specimens to the laboratory at the end of the day's schedule. An aide or an orderly may be assigned to this task. In any event, an effective system must be used to insure that all specimens reach the laboratory for processing.

Container and Labeling. Glass jars, waxed cardboard boxes or polyethylene bags serve as containers for specimens. Each container is labeled accurately with the date, the name of the patient, the room number, the surgeon, the operative procedure and the tissue to be examined. A patient may have more than one specimen. For example, in a D. and C. and biopsy (dilatation of the cervix, curettage of the uterus, biopsy of the cervix) there will be the curettings from the endometrium and a biopsy of tissue from the cervix. Each specimen usually is placed in a separate container and labeled accordingly. This is done in the operating room by the circulator to avoid mistakes or confusion as to what specimen belongs to which patient.

Fixative. A 10 per cent solution of aqueous formalin most often is used as the fixative until the specimen is processed further by the laboratory personnel. Small, difficult-to-see specimens may be placed on a piece of gauze sponge in the container and then submerged in formalin.

Cultures and smears are not treated with formalin, but to avoid drying out of cells they are sent to the laboratory immediately upon removal. When cultures are placed immediately into media, they can be stored in a designated incubator until the laboratory personnel are ready for them. Hospital policy determines the procedure used for the handling of cultures and smears.

Collection; Specimen Book. Some surgeries have refrigerators in which routine specimens are placed until they go to the laboratory. Others provide a special container or a basket in the clean-up room for specimens, and as specimens come from the surgery rooms, they are stacked in this container until they are sent to or picked up by the laboratory.

When each specimen is brought to the designated area, an entry is made in the Specimen Book by the person who places it in the special container. This entry includes the information already listed on the specimen container, plus the name of the person writing the entry in the book. There is one other column in the book which is headed "Received By." The person from the laboratory who receives the specimens checks the specimens in the container with those listed in the book and signs the column, indicating that he has received the listed specimens and the pathology sheets.

There may be exceptions to the above routine procedure. When a specimen is large, such as an amputated extremity or a massive fibroid uterus, routine containers cannot be used. The uterus, covered with a well wrung-out moist towel may be placed in a large basin. If the specimen is an extremity, it may be wrapped in a sterile sheet. With the important identification information, these specimens are taken directly to the laboratory for processing.

Special Situations. The policies of the obstetrics and gynecology department are followed in the disposal of the placenta following a caesarian section birth. Special procedures and policies often are developed in other special situations, such as saving cartilage or bone fragments for future use, or the removal and the storage of corneal transplants.

In summary, *any* tissue, i.e., teeth, tonsils, hernia sac, hemorrhoids, appendix, gallbladder, removed from *any* patient should be preserved efficiently and sent to the laboratory for evaluation and processing. It is vital that there be a permanent pathology record of the surgery performed.

CARE OF ROOM, EQUIPMENT, SUPPLIES AND INSTRUMENTS

It is customary, and certainly time-saving, for each surgery to have a routine clean-up procedure for dismantling a room following one operation and resetting it for the next patient. Each step of the process then follows an orderly fashion. The scrub assistant works with certain aspects of the clean-up, and the circulating nurse in others. The orderly has his responsibilities, and so does the anesthetist. Together the work is done rapidly, and no details are omitted.

Used linens, instruments, basins and supplies must be gathered and removed from the operating room to the clean-up area. The instrument table serves as a convenient portable carrier.

Preparation for Removing Used Items From the Operating Room

Operating rooms are equipped with a laundry hamper into which the discarded towels, linens and wrappers from used supplies are placed. Nothing is removed from the room until the end of the operation. A fresh laundry bag is used for each operation.

At the completion of the surgery the scrub assistant pushes her tables back out of the way and places the discarded drapes on top of the instrument table. While the circulating nurse is engaged in assisting the surgeon with the dressings and taking care of the patient, the scrub assistant checks the used drapes for instruments (especially towel clips, which hold the towel drapes in place) and then discards the drapes in the linen hamper.

All wrappers (if they are not paper) and all linens are discarded in the hamper, whether or not they have been used. Repeated autoclaving of linens without the moisture content that is left in the fabric when it is freshly laundered causes superheating[1] and shortens the life of the item. Unused laparotomy (lap) sponges may be sent to the laundry with the other linens, or they may be discarded, as is preferred practice. Used sponges are left in the waterproof plastic liners of the kick buckets and later are discarded with trash for incineration. Ends of sutures, glass from broken ampules, sponges from the "prep" tray, etc., likewise may be discarded.

Water from a solution basin is run through the suction tip and tubing. The tip is disconnected from the tubing. The bulb end of the tip is unscrewed and freed of blood or debris that may have accumulated; this is done with an applicator. The bulb then is replaced, and the metal tip is processed with the instruments. The tubing is disconnected from the bottle, and the bottle cap is removed. (See Chap. 7, p. 122.) The bottle, the cap, the tubing and the tip are placed on the instrument table.

Instruments that have blood or other debris on them should be washed off in a solution basin. The ratchets are opened on all instruments, and then they are placed

[1] Perkins, John: Principles and Methods of Sterilization, pp. 110–111, Springfield, Ill., Thomas, 1956.

in a tray (brought into the room by the circulating nurse) which fits into the instrument washer-sterilizer. (See Chap. 4, p. 48.) Surgical needles are replaced in their stainless steel perforated box on the rack. Scalpel blades (if detachable) are washed and placed in the needle box with the needles. Special caution should be used with scalpel blades, which are small, extremely sharp and dangerous. They are easily lost, or they may go through a perforated hole in the washer-sterilizer tray and can be the cause of injury to personnel. Blades are not reused, but they should go through terminal instrument sterilization before they are discarded. The needle box is placed with the instruments in the tray. The sponge forceps from the "prep" tray also are included.

Unused and clean 4- x 4-inch sponges are left on the instrument table and later are returned to unsterile stock to be recounted and reprocessed. The turnover of sponges is considered to be fast enough, so that superheating of their fabric is no problem.

Unused tubes of sutures are rinsed off, dried, and placed in the small tray used for the suture book (folded towel containing sutures in readiness during surgery). Glass from the suture bag (tubes are broken in this during surgery) is discarded in the container with the soiled 4- x 4-inch sponges, and the empty bag is put in the laundry hamper. Suture materials with swaged needles, if open, are discarded, because they cannot be resterilized. Unopened sutures in packets are saved and returned to the manufacturer for reprocessing.

Members of the operating room team rinse their gloves in a solution basin before stripping them off in the room, or the scrub assistant assists them with their removal. She also assists the surgeon and his assistants to remove gowns, caps and masks, which are discarded in the linen hamper in the room. Gloves used in the case, including gloves from the "prep" tray, are collected in one of the solution basins and placed on the instrument table. When the table is moved to the clean-up area, the gloves are deposited in a designated receptacle and processed as described in Chapter 5, page 82. Torn or disposable gloves are discarded in the container intended for the incinerator.

Water and saline in the solutions basins are poured out in a utility sink. The Mayo tray and basins are stacked neatly on the instrument table with the other supplies. The drapes used for both are put in the laundry hamper. Kick buckets and their contents are placed near the door of the operating room for the orderly to care for.

When these dismantling steps are completed, the labeled specimen or specimens are added to the items on the table, and the scrub assistant rolls the table to the clean-up area.

DISMANTLING CONTINUED IN CLEAN-UP AREA

The scrub assistant empties the suction bottle in a flushing hopper or utility sink, rinses it, then places the instruments, with the suction bottle, tubing and bottle cap on top, in the washer-sterilizer with appropriate detergent added and sets the automatic controls for a cycle. When the cycle is completed, the instruments are removed and either hand-washed and dried or placed in an ultrasonic cleaner (see Chap. 5, p. 68), after which they are ready for reprocessing or storage.

The suction bottle is washed and dried after it has been through the cycle. Water is forced through the suction tubing by way of a faucet attachment designed for this purpose. The lumen must be free, clean and damp inside when it is resterilized. The metal tip may be attached to the tubing, and both are reprocessed as a unit. The bottle, the bottle cap and the tip and tubing are clean and ready to be wrapped. Sterile suction sets are used for each operation.

Scalpel blades are removed from the needle box and discarded in a special container for blades only. Needle boxes are processed with the instruments.

Any specimen taken from the patient during the operation is placed in its proper container and recorded in the Specimen Book.

The basins, the Mayo tray and the "prep" tray are washed in a disinfectant solution, rinsed, dried, and then neatly stacked in a designated place, from which they are taken to be wrapped and reprocessed.

The drape from the instrument table is put in a linen hamper, and the table is washed with a disinfectant solution and returned to the operating room.

CLEANING THE OPERATING ROOM

In the operating room the operating table is stripped of linen; the table and the table pad are wiped down with a disinfectant solution (see Chap. 4, p. 62), the wheels are unlocked, and the table is moved from the center of the floor so that the orderly who cleans the floor is sure to clean under it. Any spots of soil or blood that have resulted from the operation are removed. The table for the transfer forceps, the solution basin stands, the Mayo table and the "prep" table are wiped down with a disinfectant solution. Special care is taken in the cleaning of the bases of the operating room table, the Mayo stand and the platforms.

The orderly removes the laundry bag from the hamper and replaces it with a fresh one. He takes the soiled laundry in the bag to the room provided for storing it until it is sent to the laundry by cart. He also removes the kick buckets and disposes their contents in the incinerator or in a covered container in the janitor's closet, from which they are taken to the incinerator. He washes the buckets with a disinfectant solution, dries them and returns them to the operating room. The frames are cleaned before replacing the buckets, and new moistened liners are placed in each one.

Flooding the floor with a disinfectant solution from a machine designed for this purpose, then rinsing and vacuuming it dry is the most efficient way to do the floor. If the floor is mopped by hand, a fresh solution of disinfectant should be used for each room. The mop must be clean; mop heads are sent to the laundry daily.

COMPLETION OF RECORDS

The circulating nurse completes the Surgery Data Slip and takes it and the Sponge Count Sheet to their point of collection (see pp. 170–173). This may be the ward clerk's desk or the operating room supervisor's office. The circulating nurse obtains the signed pathology sheet from the surgeon and places it in the specimen book. She then returns to the operating room.

CLEANING OTHER EQUIPMENT

Table accessories such as stirrups, foot extension, I.V. arm boards, etc., are cleaned and returned to their proper storage places. If stirrups have been used, the straps are removed and placed in the laundry hamper. Clean ones are put on the stirrups.

The anesthesia department takes care of its equipment, table and machines. The suction apparatus used by the anesthetist may be cared for by the scrub assistant in the same manner that the surgeon's is, or the aide taking care of anesthesia equipment may be responsible for its care.

RESETTING THE ROOM

When the cleaning of the room has been completed, the circulating nurse checks the position of the operating room table and makes sure that the wheels are locked, dresses the operating room table with fresh linen, and puts furniture and packs in position for setting up the next case. She then opens the packs while the scrub assistant rescrubs. Anticipated equipment needed is brought into the room and prepared for use.

REVIEW QUESTIONS:
1. What is the purpose of the recovery room?
2. Name the fixative solution for specimens that is used in your hospital. What is the routine procedure for the care of specimens and their delivery to the laboratory?
3. Discuss the importance of proper care and labeling of specimens.
4. Are cultures and smears treated the same as other specimens? If not, how does the treatment differ?
5. Describe the use of the Specimen Book.
6. What is your hospital or operating room policy in relation to the disposal of dismembered parts of the body?
7. Enumerate the responsibilities of the scrub assistant and those of the circulating nurse in dismantling a surgery room at the termination of a case.

Bibliography

Beal, J. M.: Manual of Recovery Room Care, ed. 2, New York, Macmillan, 1962.
Brown, G. C., and Prickett, E. A.: Processing of Surgical Instruments, The Journal of

Hospital Research, Erie, Pa., published by the Research and Educational Divisions of the American Sterilizer Company, July 1964.

Brunner, L. S., *et al.:* Textbook of Medical-Surgical Nursing, Philadelphia, Lippincott, 1964.

Ferguson, L. K., and Sholtis, L. A.: Eliason's Surgical Nursing, ed. 11, Philadelphia, Lippincott, 1959.

Perkins, John: Principles and Methods of Sterilization, Springfield, Ill., Thomas, 1956.

Sadove, M. S., and Cross, J. S.: The Recovery Room, Philadelphia, Saunders, 1956.

UNIT **6**

Problem Situations and Responsibilities

CHAPTER 13

MEDICOLEGAL IMPLICATIONS AND RESPONSIBILITIES

RESPONSIBILITY OF THE OPERATING ROOM TECHNICIAN : TYPES
OF LEGAL INVOLVEMENT : COMMON ACTS OF NEGLIGENCE IN
THE OPERATING ROOM : DYING DECLARATION : NARCOTICS :
BASIC RULES OF CONDUCT : HOSPITAL RESPONSIBILITY

RESPONSIBILITY OF THE OPERATING ROOM TECHNICIAN

There is every indication that, with the changing pattern of personnel involved in giving care to patients, the surgical technician will be legally responsible for his actions. The operating room technician, together with the many auxiliary workers in the hospital—aides, practical nurses, orderlies and nurse's helpers, as well as nursing students—all fall within the same category of legal responsibility as that of the registered nurse. *Each* is responsible for his or her own acts within the framework of his or her individual functions, job requirements and training.

Responsibility increases as individuals progress in their knowledge and experience. It is well to remember that anyone who assumes some nursing function becomes subject to responsibilities, and failure to perform them may constitute negligence and be subject to legal action. The following is an example. A registered nurse, not usually held liable for the negligence of others, could be so held if she delegated to an assistant or an auxiliary worker duties that could not be done without instruction and then failed to give the necessary instruction, or failed to give the necessary supervision when it was her responsibility to do so.

However, if the operating room technician is delegated a duty that his training and experience have not prepared him to do, and he proceeds to try but makes an error, resulting in injury to a patient, he is responsible for his own act and the consequences thereof. Therefore, he should make known his lack of knowledge or his inability to do an assigned duty to his immediate nurse supervisor, so that either he receives the necessary instructions and supervision, or the duty is assigned to someone capable of performing it.

If the nurse supervisor has provided instruction and supervision of the operating room technician in doing a certain task, and the technician has demonstrated that he can do it properly, the supervisor has done her job. If the technician then is assigned this same task in caring for a patient and does it incorrectly or negligently, resulting in an injury to the patient, he alone is responsible for his act. An example follows. Whenever a diathermy machine is used in surgery, the plate under the patient is lubricated with a special jelly to prevent the patient from receiving burns. If the technician is asked to prepare the plate, and he neglects to lubricate it, and his failure to do so results in the patient's receiving a burn, the technician may be held liable for his negligence. The close association of the team members in surgery probably would prevent such an occurrence, because someone probably would notice the oversight immediately, but there have been times when the error was not noted.

Since the operating room is the most hazardous patient area in a hospital, a high standard and level of performance are expected of all personnel who work there. If this standard is not met, and a patient is injured as a result, it is logical that in the future the technician as well as the nurse, the surgeon or the anesthesiologist, and the hospital can be held liable if negligence is proven.

TYPES OF LEGAL INVOLVEMENT

MALPRACTICE

Suits filed against physicians are more usually those of malpractice. Malpractice means bad, wrong or injudicious treatment resulting in injury, unnecessary suffering or death of the patient and proceeding from ignorance, carelessness, want of proper professional skill, disregard of established rules or principles, and neglect or a malicious criminal intent. A malpractice suit against a physician also might name the hospital and other operating room personnel as well, and include negligence on the part of the nurse and the auxiliary personnel.

NEGLIGENCE

The legal charge most frequently brought against operating room personnel is the one of negligence. Negligence may apply to physicians, but it is more often used when referring to the failure of the nurse, or other auxiliary members of the nursing service team, to apply reasonable and ordinary care in the application of knowledge, and to use their best judgment in the treatment and the care of patients. One definition states:

Negligence has been defined as the omission to do something which a reasonable person, guided by those ordinary considerations which ordinarily regulate human affairs, would do, or something which a reasonable and prudent person would not do.[1]

1 Creighton, Helen: Law Every Nurse Should Know, p. 74, Philadelphia, Saunders, 1957.

The hospital may become liable when it admits a patient and undertakes his care and treatment without recognizing the implied agreement or contract between the hospital and the patient. When the hospital admits the patient, it is implying that its personnel and employees possess the skills and the abilities necessary to care for the patient, and that they will use reasonable care and judgment in so doing. If a patient suffered a fractured leg because he was in a sedated condition and fell off the stretcher when he was being wheeled to the operating room, the hospital has not fulfilled the implied contract with the patient that it made when he was admitted.

If the circumstances were that it was a policy of the hospital and the operating room that all sedated patients being transported on stretchers have a safety belt in place and fastened above the knees, and all personnel engaged in transporting patients on stretchers were aware of this policy and the reasons for it, and someone failed through carelessness to comply, individual responsibility could be identified. Each person is responsible for his own acts.

However, if the facts had been that the safety belt on that particular stretcher was broken, that it had been reported, and repair had been requisitioned, but due to the limited number of stretchers this one had to be pressed into service to get the patients to the operating room on schedule before the repair was made, the responsibility for the patient's injury might be spread to include a number of people. Some of the questions to be asked might be: Who decided to use the stretcher with the broken belt, and on whose authority? Were they aware that the belt was broken? Why was a new one not available through supply? Was the supervisor aware of the broken belt? Where did the responsibility lie for the repair? Why were not adequate numbers of stretchers available for the needs of patient transportation? And so on. It could be decided that there was concurrent negligence by several people.

If the hospital had no specific policy in relation to the transportation of patients to the operating room, and the personnel had been given no specific instructions concerning precautions that should be taken for the safety of the patient, the hospital could be held legally liable for the patient's injury through negligence.

COMMON ACTS OF NEGLIGENCE IN THE
OPERATING ROOM

There are several common acts of negligence committed by operating room personnel in particular. *Causing patient falls* is one of these. Such falls may be the result of an act omitted, such as the fastening of the safety belt, or an act committed, such as improperly moving a patient from a stretcher to the operating room table.

Overlooking sponges is another act of negligence. It can result in infections, delayed recovery or even death, and it is often followed by actions for damages due to negligence. Obviously, operating room policies regarding sponge counts must be followed conscientiously to prevent sponge losses.

If any person, even one with little or no training, or a practical nurse or an operating room technician were to fill a hot water bottle with very hot water and place it against an unconscious patient, with the result that the patient was *burned,* the person would in all likelihood be deemed liable for such an act.

Faulty or defective apparatus and equipment may cause injury to a patient. This is one of the greatest dangers in the operating room, especially in the charitable hospitals, which previously have been immune from suit and have tried to continue to "get by" with using old or makeshift equipment, either because they could not afford to purchase new equipment, or because an administrator did not feel it was necessary to do so. If equipment is known to be faulty and is used in spite of this (i.e., it has frayed electric cords, broken or cracked plugs, etc.), and a patient is injured as a result, the personnel may be held liable. If, however, the defect in the apparatus or equipment is a hidden one, the law does not require anyone to know that the defect is present. The personnel using the equipment have a right to assume that hospital equipment is safe for the purposes intended, and they then would not be guilty of wrongdoing by using it.

Abandonment also is considered to be negligence. When a patient is brought to the receiving area of the operating room, and the policy states that the patient should not be left alone, the person responsible should remain with the patient. In one situation a lively 2-year-old boy scheduled for a tonsillectomy was brought to the operating room in his crib. He was wide awake and talking with the various people who came by. The aide who was assigned to stay with him left for a few minutes to get a drink of water. While she was gone, the child jumped over the top of the crib side and landed on the floor, resulting in a fractured clavicle (collar bone). The aide was charged with abandonment.

Damage to or loss of a patient's property seldom occurs in the operating room, but it can happen. Negligent loss or damage of property is based on the responsibility of the individual to act as a prudent and reasonable person. If an outpatient wearing glasses arrives for a cystoscopic examination, and the glasses are removed and placed on a table in the cystoscopic room, where later the technician puts a tray on top of them, breaking the glasses, the technician can be held personally liable for his act of negligence in regard to the patient's property.

DYING DECLARATION

The operating room technician as well as the nurse could be in a situation in which circumstances make them witness to a dying declaration. This is a statement made by a person who has no hope of recovery and believes himself to be dying, telling of the circumstances and the cause of his injury or illness. Generally, such statements are admitted by the court in cases of murder. A dying declaration may be oral, but the person to whom it is made should write it down as nearly in the patient's actual words as possible, and then read it back to the person to see if it is correct. If it is at all possible, the signature of the person making the dying declaration should be obtained, and those persons present should be asked to witness the signature.

NARCOTICS

Under the Harrison Narcotic Act, nurses have no right to possess narcotics. Narcotics should be maintained in locked vaults in the hospital or in the community pharmacy. Supplies needed for immediate use in a ward or the operating room should be kept in a carefully locked closet, with only the nurse having a key. If a narcotic is dispensed by a physician, any unused portion remaining should be returned to the physician. The operating room technician is not authorized to handle narcotics. If he were to, it would be a violation of Federal law, and he would be subject to investigation by the Federal Narcotics Bureau and prosecuted in the Federal courts.

BASIC RULES OF CONDUCT

All hospital personnel are citizens as well as employees. They are subject to civil and criminal actions just as everyone is if the circumstances warrant it. Pilfering the lockers or pockets of co-workers or the belongings of a patient, stealing hospital linens and supplies, or cheating the hospital (the employer) by loafing or disappearing on personal "business" when on duty are practices that are intolerable in the actions of an employee. It may be that when the person is caught doing any one or several of these acts, the only result is that he loses his job and must seek employment elsewhere. However, more drastic and legal action may be taken if the circumstances warrant it. It most certainly becomes a black mark on his employment record and may actually make it impossible for him to secure employment in another institution.

It should be called to the attention of all personnel caring for patients that most legal suits come from patients who have had poor results from treatment. A friendly patient who feels that all the people who have shared in his care have done their best for him is not the one likely to sue. Hence, the need for tactful handling of patients who are dissatisfied with their care and progress should be evident and recognized by all who have contact with the patient.

Observing a few basic rules of conduct that often are discussed during orientation to the operating room can contribute to the betterment of the patient's attitude about his care. These rules are simple:

Do not discuss the patient's ailments with him or try to give him personal advice.
Always be courteous.
Do not discuss other patients or physicians with the patient.
Do not express personal views about treatments or medications.

Observation of these rules in all association with patients, together with the conscientious performance of one's duty, will contribute to the patient's personal feelings of dignity and worth and enhance his appreciation of the skill and care that are being exercised for his welfare.

HOSPITAL RESPONSIBILITY

At one time charitable hospitals (see Chap. 2, p. 11) were immune from suit because of the charitable exemption given them by law. It was felt that charitable, nonprofit hospitals did more good for more people when they operated on this basis, because if they were involved in expensive lawsuits, the monies they might be required to pay in damages would deprive many other charity patients of the care that the hospital otherwise could have given them.

Today the trend away from granting immunity to charitable hospitals is nation-wide. Twenty states have abolished the immunity rule, and the remaining (except for 7 or 8) have limited immunity or have limited liability, depending on the circumstances.

No one set of factors decides the legal status of a member of the surgical team in a law suit. The decision made by the court in each case is governed by the facts in that particular case. The relationship existing between the hospital and the members of the team may be a determining factor. For example, in our country, hospitals operated by the United States and the individual states cannot be sued without their consent, because the maintenance of a hospital by a government unit is a governmental function. However, employees in a government hospital are required to answer any charge of negligence against them and to pay damages to the patient if the suit is decided in the patient's favor. The Federal Torts Claims Act of 1945 confers a general waiver of government immunity from suits for wrongs arising from the negligence of Federal government employees.

Private hospitals, organized for profit making, have been and are legally liable and can be sued by an injured patient if the circumstances prove the negligence of the hospital in relation to the care of the patient. The hospital, a physician and other co-workers could be named together as the "guilty" parties in such an action.

In the last several years a distinct change has been evolving concerning nurse-doctor relationships, the exemption of charitable hospitals, and their attendant responsibilities to the public at large. Many more suits have been brought to courts of law for settlement, and consequently a broader legal interpretation of negligence and malpractice has come into being. This trend toward making claims could be a result of many things. Health and accident insurance is big business. The financial burden of an extensive hospitalization as the result of an accident, the cost of treatment, and the loss of income while off the job encourages some individuals to try to recoup financial loss. Even though the physician, the nurse, the technician and the hospital may be able to defend themselves effectively against a charge of negligence in relation to the care given to a patient, the defense still can be costly and time-consuming if they are required to furnish proof in a court of law. It is reasonable to believe that additional factors will have future implications for legal interpretation of liability in relation to those who are engaged in giving various kinds of patient care.

In our society anyone can sue anyone else for anything, if he has the time and the money to do so. Proving the charges in a court of law is another factor. Despite the fact that each of us is vulnerable, it is prudent to do well and efficiently that which we understand and have been taught and to refuse to do that for which we are not prepared.

REVIEW QUESTIONS:

1. Under what circumstances might you be held liable for negligence?
2. Name some of the things that you can do in the performance of your job to prevent the possibility of legal action against you.
3. Would you blame someone else for a mistake that you had made? When a mistake is known, what action would you take?
4. Can a registered nurse be held liable for *your* negligence? If so, under what circumstances? If not, why not?
5. When you are in doubt as to how to proceed with an assigned task, what do you do?
6. What is your responsibility in relation to following operating room and hospital policies?
7. Under what circumstances might one be charged with abandonment?
8. What are the other frequent acts of negligence by operating room personnel, and how can they be prevented?

Bibliography

Cantlin, V. L.: The legal responsibilities of the general duty nurse in practice, Pennsylvania Nurse, Harrisburg, pp. 17–20, Summer 1962.

Cantlin, V. L., and Cantlin, E. F.: Legal facts for proper practice [a series of articles], Nurs. World 133:16, September 1959; 133:20, October 1959; 133:21, November 1959; 133:28, December 1959; 134:20, January 1960; 134:23, February 1960; 134:29, March 1960; 134:24, April 1960; 134:15, May 1960.

Creighton, Helen: Law Every Nurse Should Know, Philadelphia, Saunders, 1957.

————: Legal responsibilities of the surgical technician, Nurs. World 133:18–20, July 1959.

Hayt, Emanuel, *et al.* (in collaboration with the American college of hospital administrators): Law of Hospital, Physician and Patient, ed. 2, rev. and enl., New York, Hospital Textbook, 1952.

Lesnik, M. J., and Anderson, B. E.: Nursing Practice and the Law, ed. 2, Philadelphia, Lippincott, 1955.

Overton, P. R.: Law and order in the operating room, A.O.R.N.J. 3:65–74, January–February 1965.

CHAPTER 14

EMERGENCY SITUATIONS

MASS DISASTER : FIRE OR EXPLOSION IN THE OPERATING

ROOM : POWER FAILURE : EMERGENCIES OCCURRING IN THE

PATIENT

MASS DISASTER

Mass disasters such as multiple care accidents, plane crash, train wreck, explosion, hurricanes, tornadoes and fires present demands on the receiving and the emergency departments of the hospital as well as on the operating room. Most hospitals have recognized the need for meeting unusual emergency demands and have developed plans to meet these needs. Local Civil Defense units have assisted in this program and periodically set up mock emergencies to acquaint personnel with their roles under such conditions and to test the efficiency of plans on paper before revising them for increased efficiency.

> OPERATING ROOM PERSONNEL
> SHOULD KNOW
>
> What the disaster plan of the operating room and the hospital is. (Be familiar with the written plan.)
>
> Where emergency supplies and equipment are stored (linens, instruments, special trays and carts).
>
> What *your* responsibility is in the event of an emergency in your department.

FIRE OR EXPLOSION IN THE OPERATING ROOM

A potential hazard always exists in the operating room because gases and other combustible materials are used. Our responsibility is first to prevent such a crisis and second, to be prepared to know what to do if such an explosion or fire should occur. An invaluable source of information for every operating room worker is

NFPA No. 56, Flammable Anesthetics Code 1962,* a booklet which describes the nature of hazards, construction, equipment, administration and maintenance.

> EVERYONE IN THE OPERATING ROOM MUST KNOW
> Where the fire extinguishers are and how they work
> How to use fire doors
> How to prevent drafts and spread of fire
> How to protect patients and oneself
> The location of all exits

POWER FAILURE

A separate source of electricity must be available in the event that the usual source is interrupted. It may be necessary to rely temporarily on a battery-operated source. However, most operating rooms are equipped with an automatic switch that converts to the secondary emergency source the instant the main source of power fails. Each worker in the operating room must be familiar with the procedure in the local hospital regarding the course of action if there should be a power failure.

EMERGENCIES OCCURRING IN THE PATIENT

Many adverse things can happen to a patient which require immediate attention. In the order of priority, an emergency exists when a patient has cardiac arrest, difficulty in breathing, is bleeding or appears to be going into shock.

CARDIAC ARREST

Definition. Cardiac arrest is a condition in which there is a sudden and unquestionable evidence of the absence of heart activity. In other words, the heart stops beating. When this occurs it is a top-priority emergency. The patient can be saved by proper and prompt action. If heart inactivity should persist beyond 3 minutes, irreparable damage occurs to the brain because of an insufficient oxygen supply and an overabundance of carbon dioxide. The damage is permanent. Because of this recognized fact, resuscitative measures must be initiated immediately.

Factors Which May Influence or Lead to Cardiac Arrest. These are: insufficient oxygen supply to the brain (hypoxia), excessive carbon dioxide in the blood stream (hypercapnia), excessive amounts of anesthetic drugs, heart disease, reduced lung capacity, shock, anxiety, poor nutritional state, hemorrhage, rough handling of tissues and prolonged surgery.

Measures To Prevent Cardiac Arrest. Careful preoperative measures designed to get the patient in the best condition possible are very important. The anesthetist should make an intelligent selection of preanesthetic medications and anesthetic

* National Fire Protection Association, 60 Batterymarch Street, Boston, Mass. 02110 (50 cents).

drugs that particularly are suited to the individual patient. There must be concern on the part of all members of the surgical team to prevent thoughtless injury to the patient such as leaning on his chest, pulling too hard on retractors, handling tissues roughly, etc.

What Can YOU Do To Help in This Crisis?*

Be there! The circulating nurse must remain in the operating room as much as possible so that she will be instantly available for just such emergencies. Critical seconds can be wasted if she is not on hand.

Stand by during induction of anesthesia. Try to plan your work so that you can be at the patient's side during the critical induction phase. Keep the room quiet, doors closed; refrain from touching the patient suddenly during this state.

Remain alert! Watch for warning signs listed above. Be ready to act swiftly. If cardiac arrest occurs, immediately look at the clock to determine how much time is left, should the surgeon want to know.

Obtain cardiac arrest cart as quickly as possible. This cart should contain emergency drug supplies, thoracotomy instruments, a defibrillator, and equipment to establish an airway.

Learn and practice closed-chest cardiac massage in advance. Be ready to assist in this procedure as instructed by the physician.

Remember that time is more important than anything else—including aseptic technic.

Do your best not to panic. If you fully understand what must be done by the surgeon and anesthetist, what equipment they need and where it is located, chances are that you can be of more effective assistance.

Remember that for open-chest massage to be started, only ONE *thing is absolutely essential: a knife!* Immediately thereafter, a rib retractor will be needed to hold the ribs apart so the surgeon can grasp the heart.

Assist the anesthetist as much as you can. See that he has an emergency drug supply, syringes, and needles, and a reliable source of oxygen and suction turned on.

CARDIAC RESUSCITATION

The anesthesiologist is the key member of the team who first becomes aware that the patient is having difficulty, and that cardiac arrest is imminent. By careful recording and observing all vital signs he announces the state of emergency to the surgeon, and immediately all members of the operating room personnel act according to a prearranged plan. The anesthesiologist maintains a clear airway and provides the patient with 100 per cent oxygen either by means of an endotracheal tube or a tight-fitting face mask.

External Electric Stimulation. The surgeon may elect to stimulate the heart externally by using the electrodes from an instrument called the pacemaker (similar to the defibrillator). These electrodes are lubricated with a special paste or conductive jelly and placed on the chest wall over the apex of the heart and the upper third of the sternum (sternal notch). Between 350 and 440 volts are applied for one fourth of a second and repeated if necessary for three rapid shocks. (Fig. 116)

* Ethicon, Inc.: Point of View, Vol. 1, p. 1, 1964.

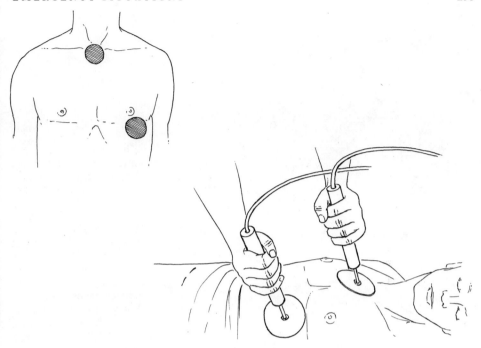

Fig. 116. Defibrillation of the heart using two electrodes. One is applied over the sternal notch and the other over the cardiac apex.

Some of the members of the team can establish an intravenous infusion for the administration of drugs and fluid replacement. Plasma, dextran and saline are typical infusion solutions and, in addition, vasoconstrictors such as Levophed (levarterenol) or metaraminol. Quinidine also may be used to reduce the irritability of the heart. Drugs are used in addition to adequate ventilation and efficient massage of the heart.

Closed Cardiac Massage. By applying pressure externally for the rhythmic contractions of normal heart muscle, circulation can be maintained at a sufficient level to sustain life. To understand the method, a review of the bony thorax will be given. The heart is limited in the front (anteriorly) by the sternum (breast bone) and at the back (posteriorly) by the spinal column. The pericardium (envelope enclosing the heart) restricts motion to the side. Therefore, when pressure is applied on the sternum, the heart is forced against the spine, forcing blood into the arteries. Relaxation of pressure allows the heart to fill with venous blood. In the unconscious patient the sternum can be pressed downward for 1½ inches without injuring the ribs. (Fig. 117)

With the patient in the supine (lying on the back) position on a firm, level surface, the person performing closed-chest massage places the heel of one hand, with the other hand on top of it, on the lower third of the sternum. Firm pressure is applied vertically about once a second. At the end of each pressure stroke the hands are

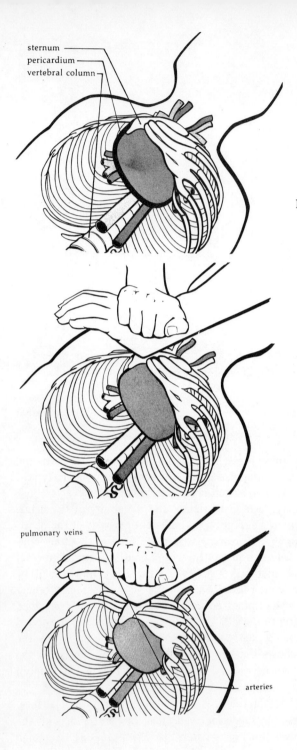

sternum
pericardium
vertebral column

pulmonary veins

arteries

Fig. 117. (*Top*) The heart is limited anteriorly by the sternum and posteriorly by the vertebral column. The pericardium restricts lateral motion. (*Center*) When pressure is applied on the sternum, the heart is compressed against the spine, forcing blood into the arteries and the pulmonary veins. (*Bottom*) When pressure is released, the chest expands, permitting blood to flow back into the heart. (Essentials of External Cardiopulmonary Resuscitation, Figs. 1, 2, 3, Philadelphia, Smith Kline & French Laboratories)

relaxed completely to allow full chest expansion. Meanwhile, another person maintains mouth-to-mouth or mouth-to-nose ventilation while cardiac massage is in progress. (Fig. 121)

Open Heart Massage. The surgeon makes an incision in the left chest over the heart. The ribs are separated at the 4th intercostal rib space, and the heart is grasped in the palm of the hand. It is pumped rapidly at a rate of about 80 to 100 times a minute. If the heart is fibrillating (quivering), the electrodes are placed directly on the heart to stimulate it. (Figs. 116, 118)

BREATHING

Is the patient breathing? A good test is to place the palm of one's hand over the nose and the mouth of the patient to feel the exhaled breath. Do not rely on the apparent up-and-down movement of the patient's chest. If the patient is not breath-

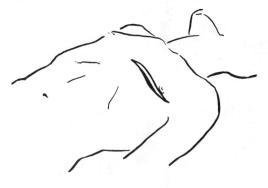

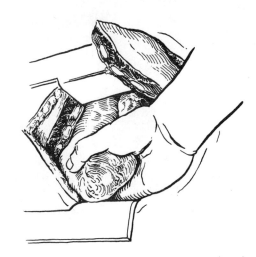

Fig. 118. Open-chest cardiac massage after incision in 4th intercostal space as shown. (Brunner, L. S., et al.: Medical-Surgical Nursing, p. 516, Philadelphia, Lippincott, 1964)

ing, first check the airway for obstruction, such as a relaxed tongue, and then if the tongue is obstructing the airway, pull the tongue forward.

Artificial Respiration. If necessary, apply.

ARTIFICIAL RESPIRATION

Clear the mouth of mucus and foreign objects.

Lift up the jaw.

Insert the fingers in the corner of the mouth.

Grasp the bony portion of the jaw and lift upward or push up on the angle of the jaw.

Pinch the nostrils to provide a closed system.

Open the mouth wide and blow until the patient's chest rises.

After blowing, turn the head to the side, and *watch* the patient's chest expansion, and *listen* to hear if air is leaving the lungs.

(Blow, watch, listen!)

Repeat at the rate of 12 to 30 times per minute.

(Brunner, L. S., *et al.:* Textbook of Medical-Surgical Nursing, p. 1152, Philadelphia, Lippincott, 1964)

NORMAL

AIR
PASSAGE
TO
LUNGS

PASSAGE
TO
STOMACH

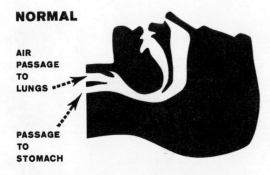

During normal breathing, air flows easily through the nose or mouth to and from the lungs.

But when the victim loses consciousness, the head tends to slump forward, and the relaxed tongue can block completely the movement of air through his throat.

This obstruction must be prevented. The tongue must be moved forward so air can reach the lungs. This step is essential before starting rescue breathing.

UNCONSCIOUS

TONGUE
AGAINST
THROAT

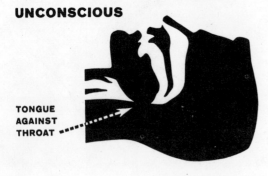

Fig. 119. Relaxed tongue obstructs breathing. (New York State Department of Health: Rescue Breathing, Improved Techniques of Expired Air Resuscitation, ed. 2, 1964)

Tracheotomy. It may be necessary for the surgeon to perform a tracheotomy for respiratory obstruction. This must be anticipated, and the proper equipment should be available. A tracheotomy is an opening into the trachea into which a tube is inserted, and through which the patient breathes. Usually, a local anesthetic is injected, but if the patient's condition is deteriorating rapidly, the procedure is done without anesthesia, since it may be most important to save the patient's life. (Fig. 122)

BLEEDING

In the operating room facilities are available to control hemorrhage. These were described in Chapter 10, page 182. For any patient in transit to or from the operating room, obvious hemorrhage is controlled by applying a pressure dressing and elevating the affected part. Since changes in blood pressure and pulse may indicate internal hemorrhage, these vital signs are observed closely. Intravenous fluids and trays as well as cutdown trays must be readily available, and the assistant needs to know how to help the physician in fluid administration. Tourniquets are applied only as a last resort.

SHOCK

A patient may go into shock (a potentially fatal condition in which blood tends to pool in the trunk of the body) because of hemorrhage, pain, prolonged surgery and

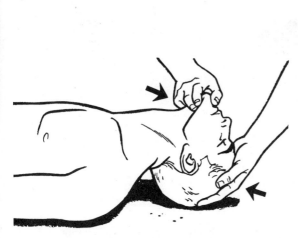

Fig. 120. The best way to prevent obstruction. (New York State Department of Health: Rescue Breathing, Improved Techniques of Expired Air Resuscitation, ed. 2, 1964)

You can prevent tongue obstruction by holding the victim's head and neck in any position which lifts the jaw and tongue forward. There are several accepted methods of keeping the tongue from blocking the throat. The most simple method, *head tilt,* involves holding the victim's head tilted as far back as you can—until the skin over the throat is stretched tight. Use one hand to hold the crown of his head firmly and push backward. Pull his chin upward with the other hand. Close his mouth during inflation through his nose and open it slightly for mouth-to-mouth breathing. Two other ways to prevent tongue obstruction are: *lift chin* up by grasping lower teeth, and *lift jaw* upward from both corners of jawbone near the earlobe.

a number of other causes. Some degree of shock is evident when a patient shows these signs: cold, pallor, clammy extremities, colorless lips, tachycardia (rapid heart beat), decreased blood pressure, apathy and thirst.

Shock can be controlled by removing the cause, such as controlling hemorrhage, relieving pain, preventing infection and minimizing trauma. Fluids are given to restore circulating blood volume, pain relievers are administered, the patient is kept warm and protected from dampness, and the feet are elevated to increase circulation to the brain.

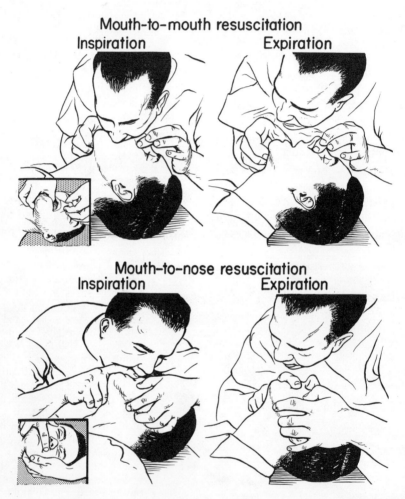

Fig. 121. Technics for mouth-to-mouth and mouth-to-nose resuscitation. (Gordon, A. S., *et al.:* Mouth-to-mouth versus manual artificial respiration for children and adults, J.A.M.A. 167:326, 1958)

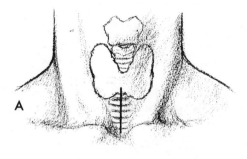

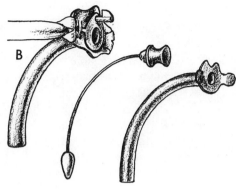

Fig. 122. Tracheotomy. (A) The incision is made directly over the trachea. A segment of cartilage is removed, and a direct airway is created. The tracheotomy tube (B) consists of three parts, the outer cannula, the obturator and the inner cannula. (C) The outer cannula with obturator in place is inserted into the trachea. (D) The obturator is removed, and the inner cannula is inserted. (E) The tracheotomy tube is held in place with twill tapes, which are tied around the neck. (Nealon, T. F., Jr.: Fundamental Skills in Surgery, pp. 179, 180, Philadelphia, Saunders, 1962)

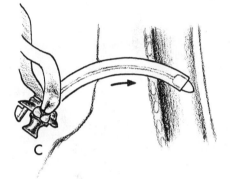

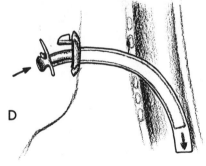

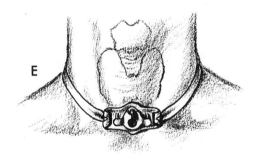

REVIEW QUESTIONS:

1. What is the emergency source of power in your operating room? How is it activated?
2. What is a simple reliable test to tell whether an anesthetized patient is breathing?
3. How can you prevent tongue obstruction in a patient? Describe ways of treating for respiratory obstruction.
4. What is a tracheotomy? Describe the purposes of the three parts of a tracheotomy tube set. How are they cared for?
5. Describe what happens when a patient is in cardiac arrest. What can you do to help in this crisis?
6. What is the purpose of a defibrillator?
7. Explain what happens to the chest and the heart when closed cardiac massage is applied.

Bibliography

Barton, J.: What would you do in case of operating room explosion? Mod. Hosp. 86:51–53, 1956.

Benson, D. W.: Changing concepts in cardiac resuscitation, Hosp. Medicine 1:15–18, March 1965.

Flammable Anesthetics Code 1962, NFPA No. 56, Boston, National Fire Protection Association, 1964.

Griffin, N. L.: Preventing fires and explosions in the operating room, Am. J. Nurs. 53:809–812, 1953.

Walk, D. H.: Are you prepared . . . ? A.O.R.N.J. 2:60–68, January–February, 1964.

Walter, C. W.: Anesthetic explosions: A continuing threat, Hosp. Topics 43:95–102, February 1965.

GLOSSARY

Abandonment. The failure to perform a duty of protecting or caring for a patient.

Amnesia. Lack or loss of memory, especially inability to remember past experiences.

Anaerobe. An organism that grows in areas where oxygen is absent or nearly absent.

Analgesia. Absence of sensibility to pain.

Anesthesia. Loss of sensation with or without consciousness.

Anesthesiologist. A person trained in the art of administering an anesthetic agent, usually a physician.

Anesthesiology. The art of administering anesthesia.

Antiseptic. An agent that will eliminate or prevent the growth of microorganisms on animate objects such as the skin.

Aqueous. A watery solution; watery.

Areola. A circular area of a different color such as the darkened ring surrounding the nipple of the female breast.

Asepsis. A condition of being without infection.

Aseptic. Without infection.

Bacteria. Unicellular microscopic plants which exist everywhere in nature.

Bactericidal. An adjective describing an agent that kills bacteria.

Bactericide. That which destroys bacteria.

Bacteriostatic. That which inhibits or retards the growth of bacteria.

Biopsy. The removal and the examination, usually microscopic, of tissue from the living body for the purpose of diagnosis.

Carbuncle. Several boils growing together to form one large abscess.

Charitable immunity. A status of nonliability for damages, or exemption to suit, given to nonprofit hospitals by law.

Chemically bound. Affinity that one chemical has with another or with other substances such as protein, etc.

Cholecystectomy. The surgical removal of the gallbladder.

Cholecystostomy. The surgical drainage of the gallbladder.

Choledocholithotomy. The surgical removal of stones from the common bile duct.

Choledochostomy. The surgical drainage of the common bile duct.

Cholelithotomy. The surgical removal of stones from the gallbladder.

Commensalism. The living of one organism on a host without harming the host

263

Conductivity. The capacity to transmit electrical charges.

Cystic. Pertaining to a cyst or sac that contains a liquid or a semisolid substance.

Cystoscopy. Looking into the bladder by means of a lighted, hollow metal tubelike instrument.

Defecation. The discharge of a bowel movement (stool).

Depilatory. Having the ability to remove hair, usually chemically; an agent for removing hair.

Disinfectant. A chemical applied to inanimate objects such as walls, furniture, etc., for the purpose of destroying microorganisms; a germicide.

Disinfection. The process of destroying microorganisms on inanimate objects.

Disassembling. Taking apart.

Dissection. The cutting apart of tissues.

Dissection, blunt. Using pressure with gauze pledget, blunt hemostat or the handle of a scalpel.

Dying declaration. A statement of the circumstances and the cause of his injury or illness made by a person who has no hope of recovery and believes himself to be dying.

Elective. As applied to surgery, the operation can be done at the patient's convenience; i.e., it is not an emergency.

Electrocautery. A wire heated to red-hot consistency; used to cut and to cauterize tissue.

Electrosurgery. The process of using high frequency electrical energy for controlled cutting, dehydration or destruction of tissues.

Endoscope. A metal, rubber or glass tube used to examine a cavity through a natural opening.

Excision. The act of cutting away or taking out.

Fenestrated. To make a hole or window into.

Fissure. A groove or cracklike opening.

Fistula. A deep ulcer leading to a hollow organ.

Flammable. Capable of burning; easily set on fire.

Fogging. The procedure of dispersing a fine spray or mist of antimicrobial solution by means of a mechanical generator.

Furuncle. A boil; a collection of pus beneath the skin.

Germicidal. An adjective describing a chemical agent that destroys germs.

Hemostasis. Control of bleeding.

Hypnosis. Artificially induced sleep or trance.

Hypoxemia. Deficient oxygenation of blood.

Hypoxia (or anoxia). Deficiency of oxygen in the inspired air.

Immersed. Placing an article or a body completely under a fluid or a solution; submerged.

Inanimate. Not alive; not animate.

Incision. The act of making a cut or a wound.

Induction. The interval between the beginning of the administration of anesthesia to the patient and his loss of consciousness.

Inert. Not active; idle.

Infection. Invasion of the body by pathogenic (disease-producing) organisms.

Inguinal. Pertaining to the groin.

Inhalation. The process of inhaling or breathing in.

Insufflation. Blowing into, as when an anesthetic gas is blown into the upper respiratory passages.
Intramuscular. Injected directly into muscle.
Intravenous. Administered directly into the vein, such as fluid or medication.

Lactation. The secretion of milk.
Legal suit. A proceeding brought in a court of law to enforce a claim or to protect a legal right.
Liability. The state of being liable or responsible.
Liable. Justly or legally responsible.
Lipid. A comprehensive term for fats and soaps.
Lithotomy. As applied to position, the legs are elevated in stirrups or leg holds to allow for perineal exposure.
Lumen. The space within an artery, a vein, an intestine or a tube.
Lymph. Slightly yellow liquid found in lymphatic vessels.

Malpractice. Bad or injudicious treatment resulting in injury, unnecessary suffering or death of the patient.
Mastectomy. Removal of the breast.
Mastitis. Inflammation of the breast.
Microorganism. Minute, living body, not perceptible to the naked eye, especially a bacterium.
Movements:
    Abduction. Movement away from the midline of the body; turning outward.
    Adduction. Movement of a limb toward the body's center.
    Dorsiflexion. Bending backward.
    Extension. In referring to a limb, the straightening out of the part.
    Flexion. Bending the various joints, such as the knee, the elbow, or the thigh, onto the trunk.
    Hyperextension. Extension beyond ordinary range.
    Pronation. Turning downward.
    Rotation. Turning or movement of a part around its axis.
        External. Turning outward away from the center of the body.
        Internal. Turning inward toward the center of the body.
    Supination. Turning upward.

Narcosis. State of profound unconsciousness produced by a drug.
Narcotic. A drug that produces sleep or stupor.
Negligence. Failure to apply reasonable and ordinary care in the application of knowledge and best judgment in the treatment and the care of patients.
Neoplasm. A tumor.

Organic. A chemical term for compounds containing carbons; pertaining to an organ or organs; pertaining to or derived from animal or vegetable forms of life.

Parasitism. The living of one organism on a host, causing it harm.
Pathogenic. Disease-producing; usually refers to bacteria.
Phagocyte. A special white blood cell capable of destroying bacteria.
Phlebitis. Inflammation of a vein.
Polyp. A hanging, saclike growth arising from the mucosa and extending into the lumen of a body cavity.
Porosity. The ability to permit passage of a liquid or a gas.
Preanesthetic. Before the administration of the anesthetic agent.

"Quat" solution. One of a large group of chemical compounds having antimicrobial and detergent properties (commonly known as quaternary ammonium compounds).

Radioisotope. An isotope which is radioactive and can be used as a tracer in the body.
Radiopaque. Impenetrable to x-ray, and therefore visible by x-ray picture.
Radium. A rare metal whose rays are used in treating certain medical disorders.
Reproduction. The ability to multiply.
Resuscitation. The procedure of reviving a person such as one who has had a cardiac arrest (heart block).

Sedative. A medication used to relax the patient and perhaps to cause him to sleep.
Spore. A resistant state or body into which some bacteria can change.
Sporicidal. An agent that is capable of killing spore-forming organisms in the free spore state.
Sterilization. The process of destroying all microorganisms by exposure to chemical or physical agents.
Subcutaneous. Injected just under the skin (used in referring to an injection).
Surface tension depressant. An agent that decreases the toughness of the film on the surface of a liquid, making it more penetrable.
Symbiosis. The living together of two kinds of organisms with mutual benefit.

Topical. On the surface.
Trendelenburg. As applied to position, the head is low, and the feet are elevated.

Varicose veins. Enlarged and tortuous veins.
Vasoconstriction. Reducing the size of a blood vessel.
Vasodilatation. Enlarging the size of a blood vessel.
Virus. A submicroscopic agent of infectious disease.
Volatile. Evaporating rapidly.

MEDICAL TERMINOLOGY

COMBINING FORMS

Root	Meaning	Root	Meaning
adeno-	gland	jejuno-	jejunum
arthro-	joint	lith-	stone
cardi-	heart	mast-	breast
chole-	related to bile	myo-	muscle
cholecyst-	gallbladder	nephro-	kidney
col-	colon	neuro-	nerve
colpo-	related to vagina	oophor-	ovary
cranio-	skull	ophthalmo-	eye
cysto-	related to sac, cyst (urinary)	orchi-	testicle
derma-	skin	os-	opening or orifice
doch-	duct	oto-	ear
duodeno-	duodenum	pneumo-	lung
entero-	intestine	procto-	rectum
gastro-	stomach	rhino-	nose
hepato-	liver	salping-	tubes
hystero-	uterus	thoraco-	chest

SURGICAL TERMINOLOGY

PREFIXES

Prefix	Meaning	Prefix	Meaning
a- or an-	without	inter-	between
ante-	before	intra-	within
anti-	against	peri-	around
circum-	around	post-	after, behind
contra-	against, opposed	pre-	before
dys-	difficulty, painful	retro-	backward, behind
ex-	away from, without, outside	semi-	half
extra-	outside of, beyond	sub-	under
hem- or hemat-	blood	super-	above, excess
hemi-	half	supra-	above, over
hyper-	higher, more	trans-	through, across
hypo-	lower, less	ultra-	excess
infra-	beneath, below		

SUFFIXES

Suffix	Meaning	Example
-desis	surgical fixation of	arthrodesis
-ectomy	removal of	appendectomy
-itis	inflammation of	appendicitis
-orrhaphy	repair of	herniorrhaphy
-oscopy	looking into with an instrument	bronchoscopy
-ostomy	incision into for drainage	tracheostomy
-otomy	incision into	nephrotomy
-pexy	fixation or suspension	nephropexy
-plasty	plastic repair of	rhinoplasty

INDEX